T0229013

Colorectal Cancer

Guest Editor

JOSÉ G. GUILLEM, MD, MPH

SURGICAL ONCOLOGY CLINICS OF NORTH AMERICA

www.surgonc.theclinics.com

Consulting Editor
NICHOLAS J. PETRELLI, MD

October 2010 • Volume 19 • Number 4

SAUNDERS an imprint of ELSEVIER, Inc.

W.B. SAUNDERS COMPANY
A Division of Elsevier Inc.

1600 John F. Kennedy Boulevard • Suite 1800 • Philadelphia, PA 19103-2899

http://www.theclinics.com

SURGICAL ONCOLOGY CLINICS OF NORTH AMERICA Volume 19, Number 4
October 2010 ISSN 1055-3207, ISBN-13: 978-1-4377-2618-3

Editor: Jessica Demetriou

Surgical Oncology Clinics of North America (ISSN 1055-3207) is published quarterly by Elsevier Inc., 360 Park Avenue South, New York, NY 10010-1710. Months of publication are January, April, July, and October. Business and Editorial Offices: 1600 John F. Kennedy Blvd., Ste. 1800, Philadelphia, PA 19103-2899. Customer Service Office: 3251 Riverport Lane, Maryland Heights, MO 63043. Periodicals postage paid at New York, NY and additional mailing offices. Subscription prices are $241.00 per year (US individuals), $357.00 (US institutions) $119.00 (US student/resident), $277.00 (Canadian individuals), $444.00 (Canadian institutions), $171.00 (Canadian student/resident), $346.00 (foreign individuals), $444.00 (foreign institutions), and $171.00 (foreign student/resident). Foreign air speed delivery is included in all *Clinics* subscription prices. All prices are subject to change without notice. **POSTMASTER:** Send address changes to *Surgical Oncology Clinics of North America,* Elsevier Health Science Division, Subscription Customer Service, 3251 Riverport Lane, Maryland Heights, MO 63043. **Customer Service: 1-800-654-2452 (US and Canada). 314-447-8871 (outside U.S. and Canada). Fax: 314-447-8029. E-mail: journalscustomerservice-usa@elsevier.com** (for print support); **journalsonline support-usa@elsevier.com** (for online support).

Reprints. For copies of 100 or more, of articles in this publication, please contact the Commercial Reprints Department, Elsevier Inc., 360 Park Avenue South, New York, New York 10010-1710. Tel. 212-633-3813; Fax: 212-462-1935; E-mail: reprints@elsevier.com.

Surgical Oncology Clinics of North America is covered in *MEDLINE/PubMed (Index Medicus)* and *EMBASE/ Excerpta Medica, Current Contents/Clinical Medicine,* and *ISI/BIOMED.*

Printed and bound by CPI Group (UK) Ltd, Croydon, CR0 4YY

Transferred to Digital Print 2011

Contributors

CONSULTING EDITOR

NICHOLAS J. PETRELLI, MD
Bank of America Endowed Medical Director, Helen F. Graham Cancer Center at Christiana
Care Health System, Newark, Delaware; Professor of Surgery, Thomas Jefferson
University, Philadelphia, Pennsylvania

GUEST EDITOR

JOSÉ G. GUILLEM, MD, MPH
Attending Surgeon, Department of Surgery, Colorectal Service, Memorial-Sloan Kettering
Cancer Center, New York, New York

AUTHORS

THEODOR ASGEIRSSON, MD
Research, Department of Surgery, Spectrum Health, Grand Rapids, Michigan

GEERARD L. BEETS, MD, PhD
Vice Chairman of the Department of Surgery, Associate Professor of Surgery, Maastricht
University Medical Centre; GROW, School for Oncology and Developmental Biology,
Maastricht University, Maastricht, The Netherlands

REGINA G.H. BEETS-TAN, MD, PhD
Professor of Radiology, Head of the Division of Abdominal Radiology, Department
of Radiology, Maastricht University Medical Centre; GROW, School for Oncology and
Developmental Biology, Maastricht University, Maastricht, The Netherlands

GEORGE J. CHANG, MD
Associate Professor of Surgery, Department of Surgical Oncology, The University of Texas
M.D. Anderson Cancer Center, Houston, Texas

JAMES CHURCH, MBChB, FRACS
Department of Colorectal Surgery, Digestive Diseases Institute, Cleveland Clinic
Foundation, Cleveland, Ohio

JAMES W. FLESHMAN, MD
Professor of Surgery, Chief, Section of Colon and Rectal Surgery, Washington University
School of Medicine, St Louis, Missouri

JOAQUIM GAMA-RODRIGUES, MD, PhD
Professor of Surgery, University of Sao Paulo; Angelita and Joaquim Gama Institute,
Sao Paulo, Brazil

JULIO GARCIA-AGUILAR, MD, PhD
Professor of Surgery, Chair, Department of Surgery, City of Hope, Duarte, California

JOSÉ G. GUILLEM, MD, MPH
Attending Surgeon, Department of Surgery, Colorectal Service, Memorial-Sloan Kettering Cancer Center, New York, New York

ANGELITA HABR-GAMA, MD, PhD
Professor of Surgery, University of Sao Paulo; Angelita and Joaquim Gama Institute, Sao Paulo, Brazil

ALICIA HOLT, MD
Department of Surgery, City of Hope, Duarte, California

JENNIFER LIANG, MBChB
Department of Colorectal Surgery, Digestive Diseases Institute, Cleveland Clinic Foundation, Cleveland, Ohio

GAETANO LUGLIO, MD
Resident, Department of General, Oncological and Minimally-Invasive Surgery - Surgical Coloproctology, Federico II University, Naples, Italy

ARNOLD J. MARKOWITZ, MD
Associate Attending Physician, Gastroenterology and Nutrition Service, Department of Medicine, The Hereditary Colorectal Cancer Family Registry, Memorial Sloan-Kettering Cancer Center; Associate Professor of Clinical Medicine, Department of Medicine, Weill Medical College of Cornell University, New York, New York

BRUCE D. MINSKY, MD
Department of Radiation and Cellular Oncology, University of Chicago Medical Center, Chicago, Illinois

HARVEY G. MOORE, MD, FACS, FASCRS
Assistant Professor, Department of Surgery, New York University School of Medicine, New York, New York

GOVIND NANDAKUMAR, MD
Assistant Professor of Surgery, Weill Cornell University, New York, New York; Former Fellow, Section of Colon and Rectal Surgery, Washington University School of Medicine, St Louis, Missouri

HEIDI NELSON, MD
Fred C. Andersen Professor, Professor of Surgery, Division of Colon and Rectal Surgery, Department of Surgery, Mayo Clinic, Rochester, Minnesota

RODRIGO PEREZ, MD, PhD
Colorectal Surgery Division, Department of Gastroenterology, University of Sao Paulo; Angelita and Joaquim Gama Institute, Sao Paulo, Brazil

IGOR PROSCURSHIM, MD
General Surgery Department, University of Sao Paulo; Angelita and Joaquim Gama Institute, Sao Paulo, Brazil

ROCCO RICCIARDI, MD, MPH, FACS, FASCRS
Staff Surgeon, Department of Colon and Rectal Surgery, Lahey Clinic, Burlington;
Assistant Professor of Surgery, Tufts University School of Medicine, Massachusetts

MIGUEL A. RODRIGUEZ-BIGAS, MD
Professor of Surgery, Department of Surgical Oncology, The University of Texas M.D.
Anderson Cancer Center, Houston, Texas

LEONARD B. SALTZ, MD
Head, Colorectal Oncology Section, Department of Medicine, Memorial Sloan Kettering
Cancer Center; Professor, Department of Medicine, Weill Medical College of Cornell
University, New York, New York

DAVID J. SCHOETZ Jr, MD, FACS, FASCRS
Chairman Emeritus, Department of Colon and Rectal Surgery, Lahey Clinic, Burlington;
Professor of Surgery, Tufts University School of Medicine; Tufts School of Medicine
Academic Dean at Lahey Clinic, Chairman, Department of Medical Education, Designated
Institutional Official, Graduate Medical Education, Massachusetts

ANTHONY J. SENAGORE, MD, MS, MBA, FACS, FACRS
Charles W. and Carolyn Costello Chair, Colorectal; Chief, Division of Colon and Rectal
Surgery, Department of Colorectal Surgery, Keck School of Medicine, University
of Southern California, Los Angeles, California

JOHN M. SKIBBER, MD
Professor of Surgery, Department of Surgical Oncology, The University of Texas M.D.
Anderson Cancer Center, Houston, Texas

EMILY STEINHAGEN, MD
Clinical Research Fellow, Colorectal Service, Department of Surgery, The Hereditary
Colorectal Cancer Family Registry, Memorial Sloan-Kettering Cancer Center,
New York, New York

SEN ZHANG, MD
Research, Spectrum Health, Grand Rapids, Michigan

Contents

Colorectal cancer (CRC) is the second most common cause of cancer-related death in the United States. CRC, however, is potentially preventable, and several strategies may be employed to decrease the incidence of and mortality from CRC. Understanding of individual risk and adherence to screening and surveillance recommendations undoubtedly will reduce CRC-associated deaths. Several natural and synthetic chemopreventive agents may prove effective for both primary and secondary CRC chemoprevention. Finally, dietary modifications (ie, increased dietary fiber, fruits and vegetables, and decreased red meat) and other lifestyle changes (ie, increased physical activity, weight maintenance, avoidance of smoking, and moderation of alcohol intake) also may lower the risk of developing CRC.

Adenomatous polyps are found on screening colonoscopy in 22.5% to 58.2% of the adult population and therefore represent a common problem. Patients with multiple adenomatous polyps are of unique interest because a proportion of these patients have an inheritable form of colorectal cancer. This article discusses the history and clinical features, genetic testing, surveillance, and treatments for the condition.

Colorectal cancer rarely occurs before the age of 50. When it does, it is often advanced and aggressive. There may be predisposing genetic and immune factors that lead to its origin. Genetic counseling is indicated for all patients younger than 50 with colorectal cancer. Before surgery, the tumor and the patient must be evaluated as fully as possible, so that optimal treatment, follow-up, and surveillance are used.

local recurrences. Laparoscopic surgery is associated with better short-term outcomes, such as shorter hospital stay, shorter duration of ileus, less narcotic usefulness and postoperative pain, and a faster postoperative recovery. The procedures are also safe and feasible in elderly patients. Hand-assisted laparoscopic colectomy is a recent hybrid technique that could reduce learning time, and its role has been established in more challenging procedures. Future prospects include robotic and natural-orifice surgery.

Several large case series and single-institution trials have shown that laparoscopy is feasible for rectal cancer. Pending the results of the UK CLASICC, COLOR II, Japanese JCOG 0404, and ACOSOG Z6051 trials, the oncologic and long-term safety of laparoscopic rectal cancer surgery is unclear and the technique is best used at centers that can effectively collect and analyze outcomes data. Robotic and endoluminal techniques may change our approach to the treatment of rectal cancer in the future. Training, credentialing, and quality control are important considerations as new and innovative surgical treatments for rectal cancer are developed.

The standard adjuvant treatment of cT3 and/or N+ rectal cancer is preoperative chemoradiation. However, there are many controversies regarding this approach. These controversies include the role of short course radiation, whether postoperative adjuvant chemotherapy is necessary for all patients, and if the type of surgery following chemoradiation should be based on the response rate. More accurate imaging techniques and/or molecular markers may help identify patients with positive pelvic nodes to reduce the chance of overtreatment with preoperative therapy. Will more effective systemic agents both improve the results of radiation, as well as modify the need for pelvic radiation? These questions and others remain active areas of clinical investigation.

Patients are not at risk of dying from a tumor that has been removed; they are at risk of dying from residual microscopic disease not removed at the time of operation. Thus, the goal of an adjuvant treatment, be it chemotherapy, radiation therapy, immunotherapy, or dietary and lifestyle manipulations, is to eradicate any residual, albeit microscopic, metastatic disease that might remain. Stage I disease carries an excellent prognosis, and at present there are no compelling data to support adjuvant chemotherapy for patients with this early stage. Stage II colon cancer also has a good prognosis after operation alone and represents the most complicated and contentious area in decisions regarding the use of adjuvant chemotherapy. Stage III colorectal cancer ($TanyN_{1-2}M_0$) represents a group at

Multimodality treatment of rectal cancer, with the combination of radiation therapy, chemotherapy, and surgery has become the preferred approach to locally advanced rectal cancer. The use of neoadjuvant chemoradiation therapy (CRT) has resulted in reduced toxicity rates, significant tumor downsizing and downstaging, better chance of sphincter preservation, and improved functional results. A proportion of patients treated with neoadjuvant CRT may ultimately develop complete clinical response. Management of these patients with complete clinical response remains controversial and approaches including radical resection, transanal local excision, and observation alone without immediate surgery have been proposed. The use of strict selection criteria of patients after neoadjuvant CRT has resulted in excellent long-term results with no oncological compromise after observation alone in patients with complete clinical response. Recurrences are detectable by clinical assessment and frequently amenable to salvage procedures.

Local recurrence from rectal cancer is a complex problem that should be managed by a multidisciplinary team. Pelvic reirradiation and intraoperative radiation should be considered in the management of these patients. Long-term survival can be achieved in patients who undergo radical surgery with negative margins of resections. The morbidity of these procedures is high and at times may compromise quality of life. Palliative surgical procedures can be considered; however, in some cases, palliative resections may not be better than nonsurgical palliation.

In 2009, the projected incidence for colon and rectal cancers in the United States was 106,100 and 40,870, respectively, and approximately 75% of these patients were treated with curative intent. Surveillance or follow-up after colon and rectal cancer resection serves multiple purposes; however, the primary argument supporting the validity of surveillance is the detection of metachronous and recurrent cancers amenable to curative treatment. The surveillance may provide some comfort for cancer survivors who can be informed that they have no evidence of disease.

VISIT THE CLINICS ONLINE!
Access your subscription at:
www.theclinics.com

Foreword

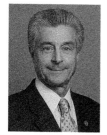

Nicholas J. Petrelli, MD
Consulting Editor

This issue of the *Surgical Oncology Clinics of North America* takes on the subject matter of colorectal cancer. The Guest Editor is José Guillem, MD from the Department of Surgery at the Memorial Sloan-Kettering Cancer Center. Dr Guillem's selection of authors has spanned the subject matter from discussions involving patients and families to lower their risk of colon cancer to the spectrum of the multidisciplinary approach of recurrent/unresectable rectal cancer.

In 2010, it is estimated there will be 102,900 new colon cancer cases and 39,670 rectal cancer cases. The combined colon and rectal cancer deaths in 2010 will be 51,370. There is no question that colorectal cancer is preventable. State cancer control plans, such as our own in Delaware that involve a statewide screening of all Delawareans 50 years of age and older with colonoscopy, has demonstrated that one can make an impact on the annual age adjusted cancer incident rates and eliminate the disparity between African-Americans and Caucasians when it comes to screening for colorectal cancer. This effort has led Delaware to be the number one state in the Country for colorectal cancer screening. Over the last two decades, colorectal cancer incidence rates have declined substantially in the United States. This decline is likely due to increased colorectal cancer screening where pre-malignant polyps can be endoscopically removed before they progress to cancer. Surgery continues to be the primary treatment for most colorectal cancer patients. Surgery can cure about 90% of colorectal cancers when the disease is found in an early stage. Advances in chemotherapy have also led to changes in treatment practice standards and improve survival for colorectal cancer patients. Although 5-Fluorouracil remains the cornerstone chemotherapy drug, it is administered today as part of a multi-drug regimen. In the advanced disease setting, targeted therapies have offered great promise in the fight against colorectal cancer.

The real key is colorectal cancer prevention as mentioned above. A major part of prevention involves the search for drugs that can safely and effectively block or reverse colorectal cancer development. I am happy to report that as of June 2010, the National

Surg Oncol Clin N Am 19 (2010) xiii–xiv
doi:10.1016/j.soc.2010.07.006
1055-3207/10/$ – see front matter © 2010 Elsevier Inc. All rights reserved.
surgonc.theclinics.com

Surgical Adjuvant Breast and Bowel Project (NSABP) has launched a colorectal polyp prevention trial (NSABP P-5). This trial randomizes patients with resected stage I or II colon cancer to a placebo tablet taken once daily for five years versus Rosuvastatin 10mg tablet taken once daily for five years. The primary aim of this trial is to determine the effect of Rosuvastatin administered postoperatively for five years on the five year occurrence of adenomatous polyps of the colon or rectum, metachronous colorectal carcinoma or colon cancer recurrence in patients with resected colon cancer. More information about NSABP P-5 can be found at the NSABP website at www.nsabp. pitt.edu.

I would like to thank Dr Guillem and his colleagues for this edition of the *Surgical Oncology Clinics of North America*. It is an up-to-date edition on the treatment and prevention of one of the most common cancers in the United States.

Nicholas J. Petrelli, MD
Helen F. Graham Cancer Center
4701 Ogletown-Stanton Road, Suite 1213
Newark, DE 19713, USA

E-mail address:
npetrelli@christianacare.org

Preface

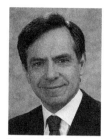

José G. Guillem, MD, MPH
Guest Editor

Recent advances in a broad range of disciplines continue to refine our management of the colon and rectal cancer patient. Due to improvements in imaging capabilities as well as our understanding of the natural history of colorectal cancer and associated syndromes, we continue to enhance our ability to tailor therapy for the individual patient and specific stage of disease.

Within this issue of *Surgical Oncology Clinics of North America*, an illustrious panel of authors addresses some of the most common and challenging clinical problems faced by surgeons dealing with patients afflicted with colon and rectal cancer.

In the first article, Dr Harvey G. Moore provides valuable information that we can offer patients and families in order to help reduce their risk of developing colon and rectal cancer. Drs Emily Steinhagen and Arnold J. Markowitz join me in addressing the challenging question of how to manage a patient with multiple adenomatous polyps. This article reviews the management of patients with multiple adenomatous polyps without a genetic predisposition as well as those afflicted with FAP, AFAP, HNPCC, and MYH-associated polyposis. Drs Jennifer Liang and James Church address the challenging question of management of early age-of-onset colorectal cancer patients.

Drs Geerard Beets and Regina Beets-Tan present a balanced view of pretherapy imaging of the rectal cancer patient including the pros and cons of ERUS versus MRI. Following this, Drs Julio Garcia-Aguilar and Alicia Holt describe the optimal management of small rectal cancers including the indications for transanal excision (TAE), transanal endoscopic microsurgery (TEM), or total mesorectal excision (TME). Following this, Drs David Schoetz Jr and Rocco Ricciardi review important technical points pertaining to optimal low anterior resection and anastomotic techniques that facilitate sphincter preservation.

Drs Gaetano Luglio and Heidi Nelson and Drs Govind Nandakumar and James Fleshman present a state-of-the-art review of laparoscopy for colon and rectal cancer, respectively. In addition to providing technical pearls pertaining to optimal laparoscopic techniques for colon and rectal cancer, these two excellent articles review the published results as well as ongoing trials addressing the efficacy of laparoscopy for both colon and rectal cancer.

Surg Oncol Clin N Am 19 (2010) xv–xvi
doi:10.1016/j.soc.2010.08.005
1055-3207/10/$ – see front matter surgonc.theclinics.com

Drs Bruce D. Minsky and Leonard B. Saltz carefully and concisely review rationale, approaches, and controversies pertaining to both chemoradiation for rectal cancer and adjuvant therapy for colon cancer, respectively.

Drs Angelita Habr-Gama, Rodrigo Perez, Igor Proscurshim, and Joaquim Gama-Rodrigues present an update of the status of the "wait-and-see" approach for patients with distal rectal cancer who experience a complete response after neoadjuvant chemoradiation therapy.

Drs Miguel A. Rodriguez-Bigas, George J. Chang, and John M. Skibber present a valuable review of how to approach a patient who presents with a recurrent or unresectable rectal cancer from a multidisciplinary perspective.

Last, Drs Theodor Asgeirsson, Sen Zhang, and Anthony J. Senagore present an up-to-date review of the optimal follow-up for patients undergoing a curative colon and rectal cancer resection.

In summary, I believe the readership will find this issue of *Surgical Oncology Clinics of North America* to be a valuable resource since it addresses some of the most common clinical problems faced by surgeons taking care of patients and families afflicted with colon and rectal cancer.

I would like to thank all of the authors for their outstanding contributions, Ms Jessica Demetriou for editorial assistance, and Dr Nicholas J. Petrelli for inviting me to edit this issue dedicated to colon and rectal cancer.

José G. Guillem, MD, MPH
Department of Surgery, Colorectal Service
Memorial-Sloan Kettering Cancer Center
1275 York Avenue, C-1077
New York, NY 10065, USA

E-mail address:
guillemj@mskcc.org

Colorectal Cancer: What Should Patients and Families Be Told to Lower the Risk of Colorectal Cancer?

Harvey G. Moore, MD

KEYWORDS

• Colorectal cancer • Chemoprevention • Screening
• Risk reduction

Worldwide, colorectal cancer (CRC) represents a major disease burden. CRC is the fourth most frequently diagnosed malignancy in men and third most common in women, with almost 1 million people developing colorectal cancer annually.[1] Worldwide, CRC is the third most common cause of cancer death, responsible for 639,000 deaths annually.[2] In the United States, CRC is the third most common cancer in men and women and the second most common cause of cancer-related death overall, accounting for 11% of cancers diagnosed.[3] An estimated 147,000 cases were diagnosed in the United States in 2009, and approximately 50,000 people died from the disease.[3]

Currently, the overall probability of an individual developing CRC in the United States over a lifetime is 5.5% in men and 5.1% in women.[4] Because CRC is a survivable cancer, with 5-year survival rates adjusted for life expectancy of 64%,[4] the prevalence of people living with a diagnosis of CRC in the population is substantial. In total, over 1 million Americans alive in 2006 have had a diagnosis of CRC.[5]

CRC PREVENTION

Several prevention strategies may be employed to reduce the risk of developing CRC. Primary cancer prevention targets individuals at average risk for CRC. Population-based CRC screening protocols are one example; others include chemoprevention, dietary modification, and other nondietary lifestyle changes. Secondary cancer prevention targets patients at increased risk for CRC, such as patients with a family history of CRC, a personal history of adenomatous polyps, or a known or suspected

Department of Surgery, New York University School of Medicine, 550 First Avenue, NBV 15-S-12, New York, NY 10016, USA
E-mail address: harvey.moore@med.nyu.edu

Surg Oncol Clin N Am 19 (2010) 693–710
doi:10.1016/j.soc.2010.06.002
1055-3207/10/$ – see front matter © 2010 Elsevier Inc. All rights reserved.

genetic predisposition to CRC. High-risk surveillance strategies, mostly involving colonoscopy, are one example. Chemoprevention, as well as dietary and lifestyle modification, also may play a role in high-risk patients, including those with a personal history of colorectal adenomas. This article focuses on primary and secondary CRC prevention: risk-reduction strategies for patients with average or increased risk of CRC, exclusive of hereditary colorectal cancer syndromes (discussed later in this issue).

SCREENING OF AVERAGE-RISK INDIVIDUALS

There is considerable evidence that screening of asymptomatic individuals at average risk for CRC can detect cancers at a curable, early stage, resulting in decreased mortality.[6–8] Although the percentage of average-risk Americans over 50 who have undergone recent screening for CRC has increased since 2005, data suggest that just over 53% of age-eligible Americans have availed themselves to available screening modalities based on a 2008 survey.[9] Although there has been a recent push to establish colonoscopy as the preferred modality for CRC screening, barriers to colonoscopy related to insurance coverage, institutional policies, and resource availability may necessitate the need for other screening modalities. Colonoscopy has never been proven in a randomized trial to reduce mortality from CRC. However, a recent population-based, case–control study demonstrated that complete colonoscopy was associated with decreased mortality from left-sided CRC (adjusted odds ratio [OR] 0.33; 95% confidence interval [CI], 0.28–0.39), but not for right-sided cancers. This may be explained, in part, by variations in quality of colonoscopy (eg, inadequate cecal intubation rate). Patients who died from CRC were much less likely to have undergone complete colonoscopy (OR 0.63; 95% CI, 0.57–0.69, $P<.001$).[10] Furthermore, colonoscopy can detect benign precursor lesions whose removal results in up to 50% decreased incidence of CRC.[11,12] Two recent studies provide strong evidence that an interval between normal screening examinations of greater than 5 years is associated with a very low incidence of interval development of CRC or advanced adenomas.[13,14] The US Preventative Services Task Force (USPSTF) recommends that colonoscopy not be routinely recommended to patients over age 75, and never for patients over age 85. In patients between 75 and 85 who have never been screened, colonoscopy may be appropriate.

Current screening controversies include the role of fecal DNA testing, virtual computed tomography (CT) colonography, and the relevance of sessile serrated polyps (SSPs). Although a detailed discussion of screening and surveillance for CRC is beyond the scope of this article, recent screening recommendations from the USPSTF,[8] the National Comprehensive Cancer Network (NCCN),[15] and joint guidelines from the American Cancer Society, US Multi-Society Task Force on Colorectal Cancer, and American College of Radiology (ACS-MSTF-ACR)[7] are summarized in **Table 1**.

ASSESSMENT OF INCREASED RISK FOR DEVELOPING CRC

The initial step to formulating a cancer prevention strategy for the individual patient is an assessment of individual risk of CRC (**Box 1**). Age is one of the most important risk factors for CRC. Ninety percent of cases are diagnosed over the age of 50.[4] In fact, as many as 30% to 50% of individuals older than 50 harbor one or more adenomatous polyps.[16] The risk of CRC continues to increase with age; the incidence per 100,000 people age 80 to 84 years is over seven times the incidence in people age 50 to 54. However, CRC can occur at any age; the incidence of CRC in patients younger than

Table 1
Colorectal cancer screening guidelines[a]

Screening Modality	Organization			Interval
	USPSTF[8]	NCCN[15]	ACS-MSTF-ACR[7]	
Guaiac-based FOBT	Recommended	Recommended	Recommended[b]	1 y
Fecal IHC test	Recommended[b]	Recommended	Recommended[b]	1 y
Flexible sigmoidoscopy	Recommended with FOBT every 3 yrs	Recommended ± FOBT	Recommended (scope inserted 40 cm or to splenic flexure)	5 y
Double contrast barium enema	Not recommended	Recommended if other tests not available	Recommended if other tests not available	5 y
Colonoscopy	Recommended	Recommended	Recommended	10 y
Stool DNA test	Not recommended[c]	Not recommended[c]	Recommended[b]	Interval not defined
Virtual CT colonography	Not recommended[c]	Not recommended[c]	Recommended	5 y

Abbreviations: ACS-MSTF-ACR, American Cancer Society, US Multi-Society Task Force, American College of Radiology; CT, computed tomography; FOBT, fecal occult-blood test; IHC, immunohisto-chemical; NCCN, National Comprehensive Cancer Network; USPSTF, United States Preventative Services Task Force.
[a] Average-risk patients (age ≥50, no history of adenoma or colorectal cancer, no history of inflammatory bowel disease, negative family history).
[b] If sensitivity greater than 50%.
[c] Insufficient evidence to make recommendation.

age 50 may be increasing.[17] When patients younger than 50 present with CRC, consideration must be given to the presence of a hereditary CRC syndrome (see discussion of early age-of-onset CRC elsewhere in this issue).

Individuals with a family history of CRC are at increased risk for development of CRC. In a recent meta-analysis involving 59 studies, the relative risk of developing CRC with one affected first-degree relative was 2.24 (95% CI, 2.06–2.43). The relative risk increased to 3.97 if two or more first-degree relatives were affected.[18] This corresponds to a pooled lifetime risk for a 50-year-old of 1.8% with no family history, 3.4% with one affected first-degree relative, and 6.9% with two or more first-degree relatives. The clustering of CRC in some families may be attributed to an inherited predisposition, common environmental exposures, or a combination of both. The influence of a more distant family history, such as second-degree relatives with CRC, on individual risk has not been firmly established.

Some of the increased risk attributed to family history is secondary to inheritance of known CRC susceptibility genes, such as mutations in tumor suppressor genes (for example, the adenomatous polyposis coli gene [APC]), as well as the mismatch repair genes such as MLH1, MSH2, and MSH6. The familial syndromes resulting from these autosomal dominantly inherited mutations, FAP and HNPCC, will be discussed in detail elsewhere in this issue.

Despite the importance of family history on risk of CRC, up to 25% of individuals with an affected first-degree relative do not report having a positive family history.[19] Those who do report a positive family history may not be aware of the associated

---

Box 1
Stratification of risk for CRC

Average risk

    Age greater than or equal to 50 years

    No personal history of CRC or adenomas

    Negative family history

    No history of inflammatory bowel disease

Increased risk

    Positive family history

    Personal history of CRC

    Personal history of adenoma or sessile serrated polyp (SSP)

    Personal history of chronic ulcerative colitis or Crohn's disease

High risk

    Hereditary nonpolyposis colorectal cancer (HNPCC)/Lynch syndrome

    Familial adenomatous polyposis (FAP)

    Attenuated familial adenomatous polyposis (AFAP)

    MYH-associated polyposis (MAP)

    Other polyposis syndromes (eg, Peutz-Jeghers, juvenile polyposis, hyperplastic polyposis syndrome)

---

increased risk.[20] These errors may be compounded by physicians who do not take family history into account when determining appropriate intervals for surveillance, despite the family history information being present in the medical records.[21] Failure to report a positive family history, recognize the significance of it, and incorporate family history into follow-up strategies greatly undermine the efficacy of screening and surveillance in preventing CRC.

Other conditions that may result in an increased risk of CRC development are chronic ulcerative colitis and Crohn's disease, as well as a personal history of colorectal adenomas and CRC (see **Box 1**). Surveillance recommendations based on family history of CRC and personal history of adenomas or CRC are summarized in **Table 2**.

CHEMOPREVENTION

Sporn[22] first coined the term chemoprevention in 1976 to represent the use of specific natural or synthetic chemical agents to reverse, suppress, or prevent carcinogenic progression to invasive cancer. A wealth of epidemiologic, in vitro, and in vivo evidence suggests that nonsteroidal anti-inflammatory drugs (NSAIDs) may be such agents. Other potential chemopreventive agents include folate, selenium, calcium, vitamin D, and beta carotene.

Aspirin and NSAIDS

There is considerable observational evidence that the use of aspirin or other NSAIDs is chemoprotective against CRC.[23] The mechanism underlying the antineoplastic action of NSAIDs is incompletely understood, but it is believed to involve both cyclooxygenase (COX)-dependent and COX-independent pathways. At least 30 observational

Table 2
Colorectal cancer surveillance recommendations based on family history and personal history of adenomas and/or CRC

	Organization	
Family History	**ACS-MSTF-ACR[7]**	**NCCN[15]**
First-degree relative with CRC <60	Colonoscopy every 5 years; begin at age 40, or 10 years before earliest diagnosis	Colonoscopy every 5 years; begin at age 40[a]
First-degree relatives with CRC ≥60	Interval recommended for average risk; begin at age 40	Colonoscopy every 5 years; begin at age 50
Two or more first-degree relatives with CRC at any age	Colonoscopy every 5 years; begin at age 40, or 10 years before earliest diagnosis	Colonoscopy every 3–5 years; begin at age 40, or 10 years before earliest diagnosis[b]
Two or more second-degree relatives with CRC at any age	Interval recommended for average risk; begin at age 40	Colonoscopy every 5 years; begin at age 50[b]
One second-degree relative or any third-degree relative with CRC, or first degree relative with nonadvanced adenomas	No recommendation	Treat as average-risk
Finding at Colonoscopy		
≤2 adenomas or SSPs; <1 cm, tubular histology	Colonoscopy in 5–10 years	Colonoscopy in 5 years; if negative, 5–10 years
3–10 polyps; ≥1 cm, villous or high grade dysplasia	Colonoscopy in 3 years; if negative or only 1–2 small tubular adenomas, 5 years	Colonoscopy in 3 years; if negative, 5 years
Incomplete or piecemeal polypectomy or polypectomy of large sessile polyp	Colonoscopy in 2–6 months to verify complete removal	Colonoscopy in 2–6 months based on clinical judgment
>10 cumulative adenomas	Colonoscopy <3years[c]; consider polyposis syndrome	Individual management; consider polyposis syndrome
Personal history of curative intent resected CRC	Colonoscopy in 1 year; (within 3–6 months if no or incomplete preoperative colonoscopy; if negative 3 years, then 5 years)	Colonoscopy in 1 year; (within 3–6 months if no or incomplete preoperative colonoscopy; if adenoma/SSP repeat 1–3 years; if negative 2–3 years, then 3–5 years

Abbreviations: ACS-MSTF-ACR, American Cancer Society, US Multi-Society Task Force, American College of Radiology; CRC, colorectal cancer; NCCN, National Comprehensive Cancer Network; SSP, Sessile serrated polyp.
[a] If <50 years, same recommendation but repeat every 3–5 years depending on other family history; begin 10 years before earliest diagnosis.
[b] Individuals should be related.
[c] Defined as >10 adenomas on single examination.

studies have been conducted to evaluate the influence of NSAID use on development of CRC. A consistent reduction in the risk of colorectal neoplasia (adenoma and invasive cancers) in NSAID users is consistently identified in these studies of various design.[23-25]

A Cochrane review summarizing the results of randomized, controlled intervention trials has been published.[26] The authors of this meta-analysis reviewed one population-based prevention trial (including 22,071 people),[27] three secondary prevention trials in patients with sporadic polyps (including 2028 patients),[28-30] and four trials in 150 patients with familial adenomatous polyposis.[31-34] The authors concluded that, overall, there is some evidence for the effectiveness of intervention strategies using NSAIDs for the prevention of colorectal adenoma. However, the single primary prevention trial reviewed[27] did not demonstrate a decreased incidence of CRC in the NSAID users. Subsequent primary prevention trials also did not demonstrate efficacy,[35,36] leading to a recommendation by the US Preventive Services Task Force against aspirin/NSAID use for primary CRC prevention in average-risk individuals.[37] However, a recent pooled analysis of two large randomized trials from the United Kingdom with over 20 years of follow-up revealed a statistically significant reduction in CRC incidence in aspirin users (relative risk [RR] = 0.63; 95% CI, 0.47–0.85, P = .002, if allocated to aspirin for 5 years or more), but only after a latency period of 10 years or longer.[38]

NSAIDs and aspirin may play an important role in secondary chemoprevention of colorectal adenomas and cancer. Logan and colleagues[39] reported a randomized, double-blind trial of aspirin and folate in the prevention of recurrent colorectal adenomas. Patients randomized to aspirin 300 mg/d had a significantly reduced risk of recurrent adenoma compared with the placebo group (RR = 0.79; 95% CI, 0.63–0.99). Baron and colleagues[40] randomized 2587 to either the COX-2 inhibitor rofecoxib 25 mg/d versus placebo. Adenoma recurrence was less frequent for rofecoxib subjects than for those randomized to placebo (41% vs 55%; P<.0001; RR = 0.76; 95% CI, 0.69–0.83).

Continued use of NSAIDs may have additional benefits. Long-term follow-up of the Aspirin/Folate Polyp Prevention Study revealed that patients who used regular NSAIDs in the 4 years following the study intervention (3 years of 81 mg aspirin/d) had a persistent reduction in development of adenoma versus patients who were infrequent poststudy NSAID users (RR = 0.62; 95% CI, 0.39–0.98).[41] In addition, regular aspirin use may result in lower cancer-specific mortality in patients with a history of CRC.[42]

Unfortunately, serious gastrointestinal (GI) complications may occur in regular users of aspirin and NSAIDs. Hospitalizations for GI complications occur in 7 of 1000 to 13 of 1000 chronic users of NSAIDS per year.[43] Celebrex and Vioxx, two COX-2 specific inhibitors, have been associated with significant cardiovascular adverse effects,[44-46] resulting in the removal of Vioxx from the US market. Thus, their use in primary chemoprevention cannot be supported.[45]

The answer may not lie with single agents, however, but rather with combination therapy. Combinatorial strategies in cancer therapy can provide dramatic improvements in safety and efficacy over monotherapy, particularly when agents differ in mode of action. In a rat model of CRC, the combination of curcumin (a nontoxic, naturally occurring polyphenol derived from the tumeric plant) and celecoxib resulted in a significantly reduced number of aberrant crypt foci compared with either agent alone.[47] Importantly, the concentration of celecoxib in that study can be achieved in people with a standard anti-inflammatory dose of 100 mg twice daily (half the daily dose associated with cardiovascular complications). In a recent randomized, placebo-controlled trial patients with a history of prior adenomas who received daily sulindac at 150 mg by mouth in combination with 500 mg of difluoromethylornithine (DFMO) for 36 months had a significantly reduced incidence of recurrent adenomas (12% vs 41%, P<.001) compared with placebo. Serious adverse events did not differ between groups.[48]

Other Chemoprevention

Antioxidants

Several antioxidants have been studied as potentially protective against CRC. These agents reduce intrinsic oxidative damage and may also inhibit carcinogenesis by stimulating the immune system directly.[23] The most promising appear to be the carotenoids, including beta carotene and selenium. Although prior intervention trials did not demonstrate efficacy against recurrent adenoma in patients treated with beta carotene,[49,50] recent data are more promising. In a prospective trial involving 864 patients randomized to receive either beta carotene or placebo, beta carotene was associated with a marked decrease in the risk of one or more recurrent adenomas among subjects who neither smoked cigarettes nor drank alcohol (RR = 0.56; 95% CI, 0.35–0.89). However, beta carotene supplementation conferred a modest increase in the risk of recurrence among those who smoked (RR = 1.36; 95% CI, 0.70–2.62) or drank (RR = 1.13; 95% CI, 0.89–1.43).[51]

Selenium also has shown promise. In a randomized, placebo-controlled trial of 1312 patients with a history of skin cancer followed for 6.4 years, patients randomized to selenium had a statistically significant 58% reduction in CRC incidence,[52] as well as a decreased incidence of adenomas.[53] However, in the recently published Selenium and Vitamin E Cancer Prevention Trial (SELECT), neither selenium nor selenium plus vitamin E was associated with a decreased incidence of CRC compared with placebo.[54] Ongoing, prospective randomized trials will further clarify the role of both beta carotene and selenium in reducing the risk of CRC.[23]

Calcium and vitamin D

A substantial amount of evidence supports the beneficial effect of calcium on the prevention of CRC. Calcium binds and precipitates bile and fatty acids as insoluble soaps, thereby preventing these potentially mutagenic compounds from contacting epithelial cells. Calcium may also directly influence proliferation of mucosal cells via protein kinase C and K-ras.[23] Two Phase 3 intervention trials of calcium for the prevention of recurrent adenoma[55,56] demonstrated that calcium supplementation (1200 mg daily for 4 years or 2000 mg daily for 3 years) was associated with a reduction of recurrent adenoma. However, only one study[55] achieved statistical significance. In a recent meta-analysis of the two studies, the relative risk of recurrent adenomas was 0.74 for patients randomized to receive calcium versus placebo.[57]

The role as calcium as a primary chemopreventive agent is less clear. Several recent cohort studies have reported an inverse relationship between calcium intake and CRC incidence, with RR between 0.68 and 0.84 in men and 0.64 and 0.70 in women.[58–61] However, a randomized, placebo-controlled trial of calcium plus vitamin D supplementation involving 36,282 postmenopausal women produced conflicting results. Women randomized to 1000 mg daily of elemental calcium plus 400 IU vitamin D for an average of 7 years had an RR of CRC of 1.08 (95% CI, 0.86–1.34) compared with women who received placebo.[62]

Vitamin D as a single agent also may have a chemopreventive effect via modulation of calcium absorption and gene expression.[23] In a case–control study nested within the Multiethnic Cohort Study, plasma 25(OH)D level was measured in 229 patients with CRC and 434 matched controls. An inverse trend was observed between Vitamin D level and risk of CRC (OR, per doubling of 25(OH)D = 0.68; 95% CI, 0.51–0.92).[63] Two recent meta-analyses investigated the relationship between circulating 25(OH)D levels and Vitamin D intake on the incidence of colorectal adenomas and CRC. In the first, circulating 25(OH)D was inversely correlated with the incidence of adenomas (OR = 0.70; 95% CI, 0.56–0.87). A similar finding was noted for high versus low vitamin D intake (OR = 0.89; 95% CI, 0.78–1.02).[64] In the second, in patients with an increase of 25(OH)D by 20 ng/mL, the OR for CRC incidence was 0.57 (95% CI, 0.43–0.76).[65] However, a meta-analysis of 10 cohort studies involving 2813 cancer cases reported that increased vitamin D intake was associated with a nonsignificant 6% reduction on CRC risk (RR = 0.94; 95% CI 0.83–1.06).[66]

Folate

Folate, a B vitamin, is critical for normal methylation of DNA. Folate deficiency may lead to CRC through disruption of DNA synthesis and repair, as well as loss of control of proto-oncogene activity.[67] Numerous prior retrospective epidemiologic studies, as well as prospective cohort studies, have demonstrated a statistically significant difference or trend toward a significant relationship between increased folate intake and a reduced risk of CRC or adenoma.[68]

Two recent prospective, randomized intervention trials examined the role of folate as secondary chemoprevention in patients with a history of adenomas.[39,69] There was no association between folate use and the rate of recurrent adenoma in either study. Of concern, patients receiving folate in one study had a trend toward a higher incidence of advanced adenoma (11.4% vs 8.6%), and at least three adenomas (9.9% vs 4.3%). Taken together, these studies demonstrate that folate supplementation is unlikely to be of benefit as secondary prevention in patients with a history of colorectal adenomas, and may actually be detrimental.

Folate may play a dual-modulator role. There may be a protective influence of moderate dietary increases of folate initiated before the establishment of neoplastic foci. Early prevention is likely due to protection against DNA damage by maintaining adequate methyl groups for DNA methylation and nucleotide synthesis. However, a promoter effect may occur on pre-established, clinically occult neoplastic foci secondary to increased provision of nucleotide precursors to rapidly replicating neoplastic cells.[70,71] Further research is required to establish the role of folate supplementation as CRC chemoprevention.

LIFESTYLE CHANGES
Dietary Modification

Fiber

Fiber is the dietary fraction that is resistant to human digestion and absorption. Fiber decreases intestinal transit time, resulting in reduced length of exposure of the colon to carcinogens. In addition, fiber may dilute or absorb potential carcinogens, such as bile salts. Finally, products of fiber degradation and fermentation in the colon also may play a role.[72] The data regarding the association between fiber and CRC risk are inconsistent. Two large cohort studies, the Nurses' Health study[73] and the Health Professionals' Follow-up Study,[74] found no relationship between use of fiber and CRC risk.

More recent studies, however, have reopened the debate. In the Prostate, Lung, Colorectal, and Ovarian (PLCO) Screening Trial,[75] a nested case–control study of over 37,508 people undergoing flexible sigmoidoscopy, people who reported the highest amounts of fiber in their diets had a 27% risk reduction for adenoma compared with people who consumed the least amount of fiber. In a second prospective cohort study involving over 500,000 people, investigators[76,77] found that people who consumed the most fiber had a 25% lower incidence of CRC than those who consumed the least fiber. In both studies, the protective effect was greater for the colon than for the rectum. A subsequent meta-analysis, involving 13 prospective cohort studies, revealed an inverse relationship between dietary fiber intake and risk of CRC in age-adjusted analyses; however, this association did not hold when adjusted for other dietary risk factors.[78] More recent cohort studies have produced conflicting results.[79,80]

Intervention studies in which an increase in dietary fiber is instituted generally have proven unsuccessful in lowering the risk of colorectal neoplasia. A meta-analysis evaluated the effect of five dietary intervention trials involving 4349 individuals in whom some form of fiber supplementation was performed.[81] There was no difference between the intervention and control groups for the number of subjects developing at least one adenoma (RR = 1.04; 95% CI, 0.95–1.13). However, a recent reanalysis of data from the US Polyp Prevention trial revealed that the subgroup of those most adherent to dietary changes (high-fiber, high-fruit and -vegetables, low-fat), defined as super compliers, had a 35% reduced incidence of recurrent adenomas (RR = 0.65; 95% CI, 0.47–0.92).[82] While the protective effect of a high-fiber diet against CRC continues to be debated, other benefits of a high-fiber diet (reduced cardiovascular disease, improved glycemic control, decreased incidence of diverticulosis) warrant its recommendation to patients.

Fruit and vegetable intake

Fruits and vegetables are a source of antioxidants, including the carotenoids and ascorbate, as well as other potentially chemoprotective constituents including the indoles and isothiocyanates. Prior studies did not demonstrate a consistent inverse relationship between fruit and vegetable intake and CRC risk. In four large, prospective cohort studies involving 427,244 participants,[83–85] there was no statistically significant inverse relationship between fruit and vegetable intake and a reduced risk of CRC.

More recent studies, however, have reported more promising results. A pooled analysis of 14 cohort studies including 756,217 men and women followed between 6 and 20 years also did not find a significantly reduced risk of CRC in the highest consumers of total fruits and vegetables, total vegetables, or total fruits. However, when examined by colon site, high total fruit and vegetable intake was inversely correlated with risk of CRC of the distal colon (RR = 0.74; 95% CI, 0.57–0.95).[86] The European Prospective Investigation into Cancer and Nutrition (EPIC) study, involving 478,732 participants, reported a significant inverse relationship between total fruit and vegetable consumption and risk of colon cancer (RR = 0.76; 95%CI, 0.63–0.91).[87]

Fruit and vegetable consumption also may reduce the risk of developing colorectal adenomas. Follow-up of 34,467 women participating in the Nurses' Health Study found an inverse relationship for total consumption of fruit, but not vegetables, on the risk of colorectal adenomas. Women who consumed five or more servings of fruit daily had a relative risk of 0.60 (95% CI, 0.44–0.81) for developing adenomas in the distal colon or rectum (<60 cm from the anal verge).[88] Another recent study compared 3057 men and women with a history of at least one adenoma to 29,413 control subjects. Total fruit consumption was associated with a significantly reduced risk of distal adenoma, whereas total vegetable consumption was not. However, high intake of certain vegetable groups, specifically deep-yellow vegetables, onions, and garlic was associated with a lower risk of adenoma development.[89]

Overall the evidence for an association between fruit and vegetable intake and the risk of CRC is inconsistent. Fruits and certain vegetables, such as onions, deep-yellow vegetables, and garlic may be protective against CRC and adenomas, particularly for the distal colon. However, given the other potential health benefits of a diet high in fruits and vegetables, there seems to be no apparent downside to advocating a diet high in fruits and vegetables to patients.

Red meat

Red meat is high in iron, a prooxidant that increases free radical production in the colon. These free radicals may result in chronic mucosal damage, or serve as promoters for other carcinogens. Red meat ingestion also stimulates production of N-nitroso compounds and other potential cancer-promoting agents including heterocyclic amines and polycyclic aromatic hydrocarbons.[90,91] Alternatively, dietary heme may have a direct cytotoxic effect on colonic surface epithelium.[92]

Three meta-analyses have been published[93-95]; the odds of development of CRC in the highest meat consuming groups as compared with the lowest was 1.14 to 1.28. A daily increase of 100 g of red meat (3.5 ounces) was associated with a 12% to 17% increased risk of CRC. The risk was substantially higher with the ingestion of processed meat in two studies (49%–54%),[94,95] but was slightly less than for red meat in the most recent analysis.[93] Taken together, the preponderance of evidence suggests that a high intake of red or processed meat increases the overall risk of CRC. However, these conclusions should be viewed with caution. Individuals who consume diets high in red meat generally consume diets low in other dietary factors such as antioxidants that may be important in reducing the risk of colorectal carcinogenesis.

Other Lifestyle Changes

Physical activity

The literature is relatively consistent with respect to the effect of physical activity on CRC risk. A greater level of physical activity (occupational, recreational, or total activity) is associated with a reduced risk of CRC. The effect is relatively small; the estimated increased risk of CRC in the sedentary ranges from 1.6 to 2.0.[96] A recent prospective cohort study involving 488,720 participants revealed that men who participated in exercise/sports at least five times per week (compared with rarely or never), had a relative risk of colon cancer of 0.79 (95% CI, 0.68–0.91, $P = .001$), corresponding to a 21% risk reduction. In women, there was a trend toward a protective effect (RR = 0.85, $P = .376$).[96] Sedentary behavior (time spent watching television/videos, at least h/d) was positively correlated with colon cancer (RR = 1.61, 95% CI, 1.14–2.27, $P<.001$) in men.[96] The effect of physical activity on the risk of rectal cancer is somewhat less consistent; some studies demonstrate no effect,[97,98] and in other studies a weaker effect is seen.[96] In the National Institutes of Health (NIH)-American Association of Retired Persons (AARP) study, there was a nonsignificant trend toward protection from rectal cancer in men (RR = 0.76, $P = .074$), but no protective effect in women (RR = 0.95, $P = .235$).[96] The amount of physical activity required to reduce CRC risk is substantial: 3.5 to 4 hours of vigorous activity (running), or 7 to 35 hours of moderate activity (walking at a brisk pace) per week.[96,99] However, for various health-related reasons, frequent moderate-to-vigorous physical activity can be recommended enthusiastically to most patients.

Obesity

Obesity may increase the risk of CRC in men and premenopausal women. Several case-control[100,101] and cohort studies[102-104] have demonstrated a strong association between a high body mass index (BMI) and CRC incidence (up to twofold increased risk with high BMI). A recent meta-analysis of 30 prospective studies revealed an increasing risk of CRC with increasing waist–hip ratio (per 0.1 unit) in men (RR = 1.43; 95% CI, 1.19–1.71) and women (RR = 1.20; 95% CI, 1.08–1.33).[105]

Although most studies have demonstrated a stronger association in men than in women,[105,106] recent evidence demonstrates that in women the association between obesity and CRC risk may be modified by estrogen. Several observational studies have demonstrated that the increased CRC risk is limited to premenopausal obese women.[103,107] In postmenopausal women, the increased estrogen production associated with obesity was thought to mitigate the risk. Not all studies have confirmed this relationship, however.[108,109]

Obesity is also a risk factor for the development of colorectal adenomas, although like the risk for CRC, the effect appears to be stronger in men than in women.[110–112]

Smoking
Compelling evidence supports an association between cigarette smoking and development of CRC. Of studies conducted in the United States with appropriate induction time, most demonstrated an association between heavy smoking and increased CRC risk at relatively high levels of smoking (≥20 cigarettes daily). A recently reported pooled analysis of the Women's Health Initiative study involving 146, 877 women revealed a significant association between cigarette smoking and the risk of CRC overall, but subsite analysis revealed this association held only for rectal cancer and not colon cancer.[113] A meta-analysis of 106 studies demonstrated a positive dose–response relationship between increasing cigarette consumption and CRC risk. The risk increased by 7.8% for every additional 10 cigarettes per day or by 4.4% for every additional 10 pack–years of smoking history. The incidence of CRC was 65.5 and 54.7 per 100,000 in smokers and nonsmokers, respectively.[114]

Smoking may attenuate the chemoprotective effect of certain micronutrients on CRC development. A recent case–control study revealed a strong protective effect of several dietary carotenoids found in fruits and vegetables, including beta carotene, on development of CRC. However, this protective effect was attenuated, or in some cases reversed, in heavy smokers.[115] Similarly, the inverse association found between fruit and vegetable consumption and CRC risk in the EPIC trial for never and former smokers was reversed in current smokers.[87] When one considers the other potentially devastating effects of long-term smoking (peripheral vascular disease, chronic obstructive pulmonary disease [COPD], lung cancer, coronary artery disease), a recommendation to stop smoking is prudent for many reasons.

Alcohol
The relationship between alcohol and an increased risk of CRC is well established. Acetaldehyde, a toxic product of alcohol metabolism, may play a role. Alcohol also may contribute directly to abnormal DNA methylation. Two recent meta-analyses of 16[116] and 5 cohort studies[117] demonstrate a strong association between alcohol consumption and development of CRC. In the first, increased alcohol intake was significantly associated with an increased risk of colon (RR = 1.50; 95% CI, 1.25–1.79) and rectal cancer (RR = 1.63; 95% CI, 1.35–1.97), corresponding to a 15% increase of colon or rectal cancer for an increase of 100 g of alcohol intake per week.[116] Similar results were reported in the second study[117] The EPIC trial was the first to look at both baseline and lifetime intake of alcohol as risk factors. Lifetime alcohol intake was significantly correlated with increased CRC risk (RR = 1.08;

95% CI, 1.04–1.12 for 15 g/d increase). Similar results were observed when only base-line alcohol consumption was considered.[118]

The findings of an association with alcohol intake are consistent; a high level of alcohol intake (two or more drinks per day) is associated with an increased risk of CRC. Therefore, moderation of alcohol intake should be recommended.

SUMMARY

Several strategies may prove effective in lowering the risk of CRC. Screening and surveillance programs reduce the risk of CRC by identifying and removing premalig-nant precursor lesions. Recognition of increased personal risk of CRC (including family history of CRC), by both patient and physician, is of paramount importance in tailoring appropriate surveillance strategies. Chemoprevention strategies may prove effective in reducing risk of CRC, although currently the risks associated with NSAIDS preclude their use except in the highest-risk patients. Combination therapy, however, may prove to be more effective with an acceptable toxicity profile. Certain dietary modifi-cations may reduce CRC risk, but additional studies are needed to clarify their rela-tionship with CRC incidence. Other lifestyle modifications, such as increased physical activity, weight maintenance, avoiding or stopping smoking, and limiting alcohol intake, appear to reduce the risk of CRC along with a number of other health benefits, and these can be recommended enthusiastically.

REFERENCES

1. Center MM, Jemal A, Smith RA, et al. Worldwide variations in colorectal cancer. CA Cancer J Clin 2009;59(6):366–78.
2. World Health Organization Mortality Datebase. Available at: http://www-dep. iarc.fr/. Accessed December 9, 2009.
3. Jemal A, Siegel R, Ward E, et al. Cancer statistics, 2009. CA Cancer J Clin 2009; 59(4):225–49.
4. American Cancer Society Website Cancer Facts and Figures 2009. Available at: http://www.cancer.org/downloads/STT/500809web.pdf. Accessed December 16, 2009.
5. National Cancer Society Cancer Control and Population Sciences Estimated US Cancer Prevalence. Available at: http://www.cancercontrol.cancer.gov/ocs/ prevalence. Accessed December 16, 2009.
6. Whitlock EP, Lin JS, Liles E, et al. Screening for colorectal cancer: a targeted, updated systematic review for the US Preventive Services Task Force. Ann Intern Med 2008;149(9):638–58.
7. Levin B, Lieberman DA, McFarland B, et al. Screening and surveillance for the early detection of colorectal cancer and adenomatous polyps, 2008: a joint guideline from the American Cancer Society, the US Multi-Society Task Force on Colorectal Cancer, and the American College of Radiology. Gastroenterology 2008;134(5):1570–95.
8. Screening for colorectal cancer: US Preventive Services Task Force recommen-dation statement. Ann Intern Med 2008;149(9):627–37.
9. Smith RA, Cokkinides V, Brooks D, et al. Cancer screening in the United States, 2010: a review of current American Cancer Society guidelines and issues in cancer screening. CA Cancer J Clin 2010;60(2):99–119.
10. Baxter NN, Goldwasser MA, Paszat LF, et al. Association of colonoscopy and death from colorectal cancer. Ann Intern Med 2009;150(1):1–8.

11. Winawer SJ, Zauber AG, Ho MN, et al. Prevention of colorectal cancer by colonoscopic polypectomy. The National Polyp Study Workgroup. N Engl J Med 1993;329(27):1977–81.

12. Lieberman DA. Clinical practice. Screening for colorectal cancer. N Engl J Med 2009;361(12):1179–87.

13. Imperiale TF, Glowinski EA, Lin-Cooper C, et al. Five-year risk of colorectal neoplasia after negative screening colonoscopy. N Engl J Med 2008;359(12): 1218–24.

14. Lieberman DA, Weiss DG, Harford WV, et al. Five-year colon surveillance after screening colonoscopy. Gastroenterology 2007;133(4):1077–85.

15. Burt RW, Barthel JS, Dunn KB, et al. NCCN clinical practice guidelines in oncology. Colorectal cancer screening. J Natl Compr Canc Netw 2010;8(1):8–61.

16. Schatzkin A, Freedman LS, Dawsey SM, et al. Interpreting precursor studies: what polyp trials tell us about large-bowel cancer. J Natl Cancer Inst 1994; 86(14):1053–7.

17. O'Connell JB, Maggard MA, Liu JH, et al. Rates of colon and rectal cancers are increasing in young adults. Am Surg 2003;69(10):866–72.

18. Butterworth AS, Higgins JP, Pharoah P. Relative and absolute risk of colorectal cancer for individuals with a family history: a meta-analysis. Eur J Cancer 2006;42(2):216–27.

19. Glanz K, Grove J, Le Marchand L, et al. Underreporting of family history of colon cancer: correlates and implications. Cancer Epidemiol Biomarkers Prev 1999; 8(7):635–9.

20. Rubin DT, Gandhi RK, Hetzel JT, et al. Do colorectal cancer patients understand that their family is at risk? Dig Dis Sci 2009;54(11):2473–83.

21. Butterly LF, Goodrich M, Onega T, et al. Improving the quality of colorectal cancer screening: assessment of familial risk. Dig Dis Sci 2010;55(3):754–60.

22. Sporn MB. Approaches to prevention of epithelial cancer during the preneoplastic period. Cancer Res 1976;36:2699–702.

23. Hawk ET, Umar A, Viner JL. Colorectal cancer chemoprevention—an overview of the science. Gastroenterology 2004;126(5):1423–47.

24. Garcia Rodriguez LA, Huerta-Alvarez C. Reduced incidence of colorectal adenoma among long-term users of nonsteroidal antiinflammatory drugs: a pooled analysis of published studies and a new population-based study. Epidemiology 2000;11(4):376–81.

25. Garcia-Rodriguez LA, Huerta-Alvarez C. Reduced risk of colorectal cancer among long-term users of aspirin and nonaspirin nonsteroidal antiinflammatory drugs. Epidemiology 2001;12(1):88–93.

26. Asano TK, McLeod RS. Non steroidal anti-inflammatory drugs (NSAID) and Aspirin for preventing colorectal adenomas and carcinomas. Cochrane Database Syst Rev 2004;2:CD004079.

27. Gann PH, Manson JE, Glynn RJ, et al. Low-dose aspirin and incidence of colorectal tumors in a randomized trial. J Natl Cancer Inst 1993;85(15):1220–4.

28. Baron JA, Cole BF, Sandler RS, et al. A randomized trial of aspirin to prevent colorectal adenomas. N Engl J Med 2003;348(10):891–9.

29. Sandler RS, Halabi S, Baron JA, et al. A randomized trial of aspirin to prevent colorectal adenomas in patients with previous colorectal cancer. N Engl J Med 2003;348(10):883–90.

30. Benamouzig R, Deyra J, Martin A, et al. Daily soluble aspirin and prevention of colorectal adenoma recurrence: one-year results of the APACC trial. Gastroenterology 2003;125(2):328–36.

31. Giardiello FM, Hamilton SR, Krush AJ, et al. Treatment of colonic and rectal adenomas with sulindac in familial adenomatous polyposis. N Engl J Med 1993;328(18):1313–6.

32. Giardiello FM, Yang VW, Hylind LM, et al. Primary chemoprevention of familial adenomatous polyposis with sulindac. N Engl J Med 2002;346(14):1054–9.

33. Labayle D, Fischer D, Vielh P, et al. Sulindac causes regression of rectal polyps in familial adenomatous polyposis. Gastroenterology 1991;101(3):635–9.

34. Steinbach G, Lynch PM, Phillips RK, et al. The effect of celecoxib, a cyclooxyge-nase-2 inhibitor, in familial adenomatous polyposis. N Engl J Med 2000;342(26):1946–52.

35. Cook NR, Lee IM, Gaziano JM, et al. Low-dose aspirin in the primary prevention of cancer: the Women's Health Study: a randomized controlled trial. JAMA 2005;294(1):47–55.

36. Sturmer T, Glynn RJ, Lee IM, et al. Aspirin use and colorectal cancer: post-trial follow-up data from the Physicians' Health Study. Ann Intern Med 1998;128(9):713–20.

37. Dube C, Rostom A, Lewin G, et al. The use of aspirin for primary prevention of colorectal cancer: a systematic review prepared for the U.S. Preventive Services Task Force. Ann Intern Med 2007;146(5):365–75.

38. Flossmann E, Rothwell PM. Effect of aspirin on long-term risk of colorectal cancer: consistent evidence from randomised and observational studies. Lancet 2007;369(9573):1603–13.

39. Logan RF, Grainge MJ, Shepherd VC, et al. Aspirin and folic acid for the prevention of recurrent colorectal adenomas. Gastroenterology 2008;134(1):29–38.

40. Baron JA, Sandler RS, Bresalier RS, et al. A randomized trial of rofecoxib for the chemoprevention of colorectal adenomas. Gastroenterology 2006;131(6):1674–82.

41. Grau MV, Sandler RS, McKeown-Eyssen G, et al. Nonsteroidal anti-inflammatory drug use after 3 years of aspirin use and colorectal adenoma risk: observational follow-up of a randomized study. J Natl Cancer Inst 2009;101(4):267–76.

42. Chan AT, Ogino S, Fuchs CS. Aspirin use and survival after diagnosis of colorectal cancer. JAMA 2009;302(6):649–58.

43. Wolfe MM, Lichtenstein DR, Singh G. Gastrointestinal toxicity of nonsteroidal antiinflammatory drugs. N Engl J Med 1999;340(24):1888–99.

44. Kelloff GJ, Lippman SM, Dannenberg AJ, et al. Progress in chemoprevention drug development: the promise of molecular biomarkers for prevention of intra-epithelial neoplasia and cancer–a plan to move forward. Clin Cancer Res 2006;12(12):3661–97.

45. Bresalier RS, Sandler RS, Quan H, et al. Cardiovascular events associated with rofecoxib in a colorectal adenoma chemoprevention trial. N Engl J Med 2005;352(11):1092–102.

46. Solomon SD, McMurray JJ, Pfeffer MA, et al. Cardiovascular risk associated with celecoxib in a clinical trial for colorectal adenoma prevention. N Engl J Med 2005;352(11):1071–80.

47. Shpitz B, Giladi N, Sagiv E, et al. Celecoxib and curcumin additively inhibit the growth of colorectal cancer in a rat model. Digestion 2006;74(3–4):140–4.

48. Meyskens FL Jr, McLaren CE, Pelot D, et al. Difluoromethylornithine plus sulindac for the prevention of sporadic colorectal adenomas: a randomized placebo-controlled, double-blind trial. Cancer Prev Res (Phila Pa) 2008;1(1):32–8.

49. Greenberg ER, Baron JA, Tosteson TD, et al. A clinical trial of antioxidant vitamins to prevent colorectal adenoma. Polyp Prevention Study Group. N Engl J Med 1994;331(3):141–7.

50. Albanes D, Malila N, Taylor PR, et al. Effects of supplemental alpha-tocopherol and beta-carotene on colorectal cancer: results from a controlled trial (Finland). Cancer Causes Control 2000;11(3):197–205.
51. Baron JA, Cole BF, Mott L, et al. Neoplastic and antineoplastic effects of beta-carotene on colorectal adenoma recurrence: results of a randomized trial. J Natl Cancer Inst 2003;95(10):717–22.
52. Clark LC, Combs GF Jr, Turnbull BW, et al. Effects of selenium supplementation for cancer prevention in patients with carcinoma of the skin. A randomized controlled trial. Nutritional Prevention of Cancer Study Group. JAMA 1996; 276(24):1957–63.
53. Reid ME, Duffield-Lillico AJ, Sunga A, et al. Selenium supplementation and colorectal adenomas: an analysis of the nutritional prevention of cancer trial. Int J Cancer 2006;118(7):1777–81.
54. Lippman SM, Klein EA, Goodman PJ, et al. Effect of selenium and vitamin E on risk of prostate cancer and other cancers: the Selenium and Vitamin E Cancer Prevention Trial (SELECT). JAMA 2009;301(1):39–51.
55. Baron JA, Beach M, Mandel JS, et al. Calcium supplements for the prevention of colorectal adenomas. Calcium Polyp Prevention Study Group. N Engl J Med 1999;340(2):101–7.
56. Bonithon-Kopp C, Kronborg O, Giacosa A, et al. Calcium and fibre supplementation in prevention of colorectal adenoma recurrence: a randomised intervention trial. European Cancer Prevention Organisation Study Group. Lancet 2000;356(9238):1300–6.
57. Weingarten MA, Zalmanovici A, Yaphe J. Dietary calcium supplementation for preventing colorectal cancer and adenomatous polyps. Cochrane Database Syst Rev 2008;1:CD003548.
58. Ishihara J, Inoue M, Iwasaki M, et al. Dietary calcium, vitamin D, and the risk of colorectal cancer. Am J Clin Nutr 2008;88(6):1576–83.
59. Larsson SC, Bergkvist L, Rutegard J, et al. Calcium and dairy food intakes are inversely associated with colorectal cancer risk in the Cohort of Swedish Men. Am J Clin Nutr 2006;83(3):667–73 [quiz: 728–9].
60. Park Y, Leitzmann MF, Subar AF, et al. Dairy food, calcium, and risk of cancer in the NIH-AARP Diet and Health Study. Arch Intern Med 2009;169(4):391–401.
61. Park SY, Murphy SP, Wilkens LR, et al. Calcium and vitamin D intake and risk of colorectal cancer: the Multiethnic Cohort Study. Am J Epidemiol 2007;165(7): 784–93.
62. Wactawski-Wende J, Kotchen JM, Anderson GL, et al. Calcium plus vitamin D supplementation and the risk of colorectal cancer. N Engl J Med 2006;354(7): 684–96.
63. Woolcott CG, Wilkens LR, Nomura AM, et al. Plasma 25-hydroxyvitamin D levels and the risk of colorectal cancer: the multiethnic cohort study. Cancer Epidemiol Biomarkers Prev 2010;19(1):130–4.
64. Wei MY, Garland CF, Gorham ED, et al. Vitamin D and prevention of colorectal adenoma: a meta-analysis. Cancer Epidemiol Biomarkers Prev 2008;17(11): 2958–69.
65. Yin L, Grandi N, Raum E, et al. Meta-analysis: longitudinal studies of serum vitamin D and colorectal cancer risk. Aliment Pharmacol Ther 2009;30(2): 113–25.
66. Huncharek M, Muscat J, Kupelnick B. Colorectal cancer risk and dietary intake of calcium, vitamin D, and dairy products: a meta-analysis of 26,335 cases from 60 observational studies. Nutr Cancer 2009;61(1):47–69.

67. Kim YI. Folate, colorectal carcinogenesis, and DNA methylation: lessons from animal studies. Environ Mol Mutagen 2004;44(1):10–25.
68. Kim YI. Role of folate in colon cancer development and progression. J Nutr 2003;133:3731S–9S.
69. Cole BF, Baron JA, Sandler RS, et al. Folic acid for the prevention of colorectal adenomas: a randomized clinical trial. JAMA 2007;297(21):2351–9.
70. Ulrich CM, Potter JD. Folate and cancer–timing is everything. JAMA 2007; 297(21):2408–9.
71. Luebeck EG, Moolgavkar SH, Liu AY, et al. Does folic acid supplementation prevent or promote colorectal cancer? Results from model-based predictions. Cancer Epidemiol Biomarkers Prev 2008;17(6):1360–7.
72. Sengupta S, Tjandra JJ, Gibson PR. Dietary fiber and colorectal neoplasia. Dis Colon Rectum 2001;44(7):1016–33.
73. Fuchs CS, Giovannucci EL, Colditz GA, et al. Dietary fiber and the risk of colorectal cancer and adenoma in women. N Engl J Med 1999;340(3):169–76.
74. Giovannucci E, Rimm EB, Stampfer MJ, et al. Intake of fat, meat, and fiber in relation to risk of colon cancer in men. Cancer Res 1994;54(9):2390–7.
75. Peters U, Sinha R, Chatterjee N, et al. Dietary fibre and colorectal adenoma in a colorectal cancer early detection programme. Lancet 2003;361(9368):1491–5.
76. Bingham SA, Day NE, Luben R, et al. Dietary fibre in food and protection against colorectal cancer in the European Prospective Investigation into Cancer and Nutrition (EPIC): an observational study. Lancet 2003;361(9368):1496–501.
77. Bingham SA, Norat T, Moskal A, et al. Is the association with fiber from foods in colorectal cancer confounded by folate intake? Cancer Epidemiol Biomarkers Prev 2005;14(6):1552–6.
78. Park Y, Hunter DJ, Spiegelman D, et al. Dietary fiber intake and risk of colorectal cancer: a pooled analysis of prospective cohort studies. JAMA 2005;294(22): 2849–57.
79. Schatzkin A, Mouw T, Park Y, et al. Dietary fiber and whole-grain consumption in relation to colorectal cancer in the NIH-AARP Diet and Health Study. Am J Clin Nutr 2007;85(5):1353–60.
80. Wakai K, Date C, Fukui M, et al. Dietary fiber and risk of colorectal cancer in the Japan collaborative cohort study. Cancer Epidemiol Biomarkers Prev 2007; 16(4):668–75.
81. Asano T, McLeod RS. Dietary fibre for the prevention of colorectal adenomas and carcinomas. Cochrane Database Syst Rev 2002;2:CD003430.
82. Sansbury LB, Wanke K, Albert PS, et al. The effect of strict adherence to a high-fiber, high-fruit and -vegetable, and low-fat eating pattern on adenoma recurrence. Am J Epidemiol 2009;170(5):576–84.
83. Michels KB, Edward G, Joshipura KJ, et al. Prospective study of fruit and vegetable consumption and incidence of colon and rectal cancers. J Natl Cancer Inst 2000;92(21):1740–52.
84. Voorrips LE, Goldbohm RA, van Poppel G, et al. Vegetable and fruit consumption and risks of colon and rectal cancer in a prospective cohort study: the Netherlands Cohort Study on Diet and Cancer. Am J Epidemiol 2000;152(11):1081–92.
85. McCullough ML, Robertson AS, Chao A, et al. A prospective study of whole grains, fruits, vegetables and colon cancer risk. Cancer Causes Control 2003; 14(10):959–70.
86. Koushik A, Hunter DJ, Spiegelman D, et al. Fruits, vegetables, and colon cancer risk in a pooled analysis of 14 cohort studies. J Natl Cancer Inst 2007;99(19): 1471–83.

87. van Duijnhoven FJ, Bueno-De-Mesquita HB, Ferrari P, et al. Fruit, vegetables, and colorectal cancer risk: the European Prospective Investigation into Cancer and Nutrition. Am J Clin Nutr 2009;89(5):1441–52.

88. Michels KB, Giovannucci E, Chan AT, et al. Fruit and vegetable consumption and colorectal adenomas in the Nurses' Health Study. Cancer Res 2006; 66(7):3942–53.

89. Millen AE, Subar AF, Graubard BI, et al. Fruit and vegetable intake and prevalence of colorectal adenoma in a cancer screening trial. Am J Clin Nutr 2007; 86(6):1754–64.

90. de Kok TM, van Maanen JM. Evaluation of fecal mutagenicity and colorectal cancer risk. Mutat Res 2000;463(1):53–101.

91. Bingham SA, Pignatelli B, Pollock JR, et al. Does increased endogenous formation of N-nitroso compounds in the human colon explain the association between red meat and colon cancer? Carcinogenesis 1996;17(3):515–23.

92. de Vogel J, van-Eck WB, Sesink AL, et al. Dietary heme injures surface epithelium resulting in hyperproliferation, inhibition of apoptosis and crypt hyperplasia in rat colon. Carcinogenesis 2008;29(2):398–403.

93. Larsson SC, Wolk A. Meat consumption and risk of colorectal cancer: a meta-analysis of prospective studies. Int J Cancer 2006;119(11):2657–64.

94. Sandhu MS, White IR, McPherson K. Systematic review of the prospective cohort studies on meat consumption and colorectal cancer risk: a meta-analytical approach. Cancer Epidemiol Biomarkers Prev 2001;10(5):439–46.

95. Norat T, Lukanova A, Ferrari P, et al. Meat consumption and colorectal cancer risk: dose-response meta-analysis of epidemiological studies. Int J Cancer 2002;98(2):241–56.

96. Howard RA, Freedman DM, Park Y, et al. Physical activity, sedentary behavior, and the risk of colon and rectal cancer in the NIH-AARP Diet and Health Study. Cancer Causes Control 2008;19(9):939–53.

97. Samad AK, Taylor RS, Marshall T, et al. A meta-analysis of the association of physical activity with reduced risk of colorectal cancer. Colorectal Dis 2005; 7(3):204–13.

98. Harriss DJ, Atkinson G, Batterham A, et al. Lifestyle factors and colorectal cancer risk (2): a systematic review and meta-analysis of associations with leisure time physical activity. Colorectal Dis 2009;11(7):689–701.

99. Slattery ML. Physical activity and colorectal cancer. Sports Med 2004;34(4): 239–52.

100. Caan BJ, Coates AO, Slattery ML, et al. Body size and the risk of colon cancer in a large case–control study. Int J Obes Relat Metab Disord 1998; 22(2):178–84.

101. Kune GA, Kune S, Watson LF. Body weight and physical activity as predictors of colorectal cancer risk. Nutr Cancer 1990;13(1–2):9–17.

102. Lin J, Zhang SM, Cook NR, et al. Body mass index and risk of colorectal cancer in women (United States). Cancer Causes Control 2004;15(6):581–9.

103. Reeves GK, Pirie K, Beral V, et al. Cancer incidence and mortality in relation to body mass index in the Million Women Study: cohort study. BMJ 2007;335 (7630):1134.

104. Sturmer T, Buring JE, Lee IM, et al. Metabolic abnormalities and risk for colorectal cancer in the physicians' health study. Cancer Epidemiol Biomarkers Prev 2006;15(12):2391–7.

105. Larsson SC, Wolk A. Obesity and colon and rectal cancer risk: a meta-analysis of prospective studies. Am J Clin Nutr 2007;86(3):556–65.

106. Moghaddam AA, Woodward M, Huxley R. Obesity and risk of colorectal cancer: a meta-analysis of 31 studies with 70,000 events. Cancer Epidemiol Biomarkers Prev 2007;16(12):2533–47.

107. Slattery ML, Ballard-Barbash R, Edwards S, et al. Body mass index and colon cancer: an evaluation of the modifying effects of estrogen (United States). Cancer Causes Control 2003;14(1):75–84.

108. Wang Y, Jacobs EJ, Teras LR, et al. Lack of evidence for effect modification by estrogen of association between body mass index and colorectal cancer risk among postmenopausal women. Cancer Causes Control 2007;18(8):793–9.

109. Hoffmeister M, Raum E, Winter J, et al. Hormone replacement therapy, body mass, and the risk of colorectal cancer among postmenopausal women from Germany. Br J Cancer 2007;97(11):1486–92.

110. Kim Y, Kim Y, Lee S. An association between colonic adenoma and abdominal obesity: a cross-sectional study. BMC Gastroenterol 2009;9:4.

111. Jacobs ET, Ahnen DJ, Ashbeck EL, et al. Association between body mass index and colorectal neoplasia at follow-up colonoscopy: a pooling study. Am J Epidemiol 2009;169(6):657–66.

112. Jacobs ET, Martinez ME, Alberts DS, et al. Association between body size and colorectal adenoma recurrence. Clin Gastroenterol Hepatol 2007;5(8):982–90.

113. Paskett ED, Reeves KW, Rohan TE, et al. Association between cigarette smoking and colorectal cancer in the Women's Health Initiative. J Natl Cancer Inst 2007;99(22):1729–35.

114. Botteri E, Iodice S, Bagnardi V, et al. Smoking and colorectal cancer: a meta-analysis. JAMA 2008;300(23):2765–78.

115. Chaiter Y, Gruber SB, Ben-Amotz A, et al. Smoking attenuates the negative association between carotenoids consumption and colorectal cancer risk. Cancer Causes Control 2009;20(8):1327–38.

116. Moskal A, Norat T, Ferrari P, et al. Alcohol intake and colorectal cancer risk: a dose-response meta-analysis of published cohort studies. Int J Cancer 2007;120(3):664–71.

117. Mizoue T, Inoue M, Wakai K, et al. Alcohol drinking and colorectal cancer in Japanese: a pooled analysis of results from five cohort studies. Am J Epidemiol 2008;167(12):1397–406.

118. Ferrari P, Jenab M, Norat T, et al. Lifetime and baseline alcohol intake and risk of colon and rectal cancers in the European prospective investigation into cancer and nutrition (EPIC). Int J Cancer 2007;121(9):2065–72.

How to Manage a Patient with Multiple Adenomatous Polyps

Emily Steinhagen, MD[a], Arnold J. Markowitz, MD[b,c],
José G. Guillem, MD, MPH[a,d],*

KEYWORDS

- Polyposis • Familial adenomatous polyposis
- Attenuated familial adenomatous polyposis • Lynch syndrome
- MUTYH-associated polyposis
- Familial colorectal cancer syndrome X

Adenomatous polyps are found on screening colonoscopy in 22.5% to 58.2% of the adult population and therefore represent a common problem.[1] Patients with multiple adenomatous polyps are of unique interest because a proportion of these patients have an inheritable form of colorectal cancer.

Patients with adenomatous polyps are categorized into 6 groups. The first 2 groups are autosomal dominant syndromes, namely, familial adenomatous polyposis (FAP) and its less virulent subtype, attenuated FAP (AFAP). The third group is Lynch syndrome, which is also transmitted in an autosomal dominant fashion and caused by a mutation in a mismatch repair (MMR) gene. Another group is familial colorectal cancer syndrome X (FCC X), which includes patients with a strong family history of colorectal cancer, also transmitted in an apparent autosomal dominant fashion, but who do not have a detectable mutation. The fifth group, MUTYH-associated polyposis (MAP), is transmitted in an autosomal recessive manner and is caused by mutations in the MUTYH gene. Some patients may not meet the criteria for a known polyposis syndrome

The authors have nothing to disclose.

[a] Colorectal Service, Department of Surgery, The Hereditary Colorectal Cancer Family Registry, Memorial Sloan-Kettering Cancer Center, 1275 York Avenue, C-1077, New York, NY 10065, USA

[b] Gastroenterology and Nutrition Service, Department of Medicine, The Hereditary Colorectal Cancer Family Registry, Memorial Sloan-Kettering Cancer Center, 1275 York Avenue, H 505, New York, NY 10065, USA

[c] Department of Medicine, Weill Medical College of Cornell University, New York, NY 10065, USA

[d] Department of Surgery, Weill Cornell Medical College of Cornell University, New York, NY 10065, USA

* Corresponding author. Colorectal Service, Department of Surgery, The Hereditary Colorectal Cancer Family Registry, Memorial Sloan-Kettering Cancer Center, 1275 York Avenue, C-1077, New York, NY 10065.

E-mail address: guillemj@mskcc.org

and may not have a detectable mutation but nevertheless present with multiple adenomatous polyps. In this article, the authors review the presentation, options for genetic testing, surveillance recommendations, medical therapies, and timing and choice of surgical procedures for patients with multiple adenomatous polyps.

HISTORY AND CLINICAL FEATURES

Patients with multiple adenomatous polyps may be asymptomatic. Alternatively, they may present with abdominal pain, rectal bleeding, anemia, mucous discharge, or a change in bowel habits as a result of polyps or a colorectal cancer. Patients may also present because of a known family history of polyps or colorectal cancer. A detailed personal and family history taking along with a careful physical examination may reveal other features suggestive of a polyposis syndrome.

A complete colonoscopy of the cecum with adequate bowel preparation is essential for the accurate determination of polyp burden and distribution. The size, number, and distribution of polyps should be noted, and their histopathology carefully reviewed. Hamartomatous and hyperplastic polyposis should be ruled out because patients with these conditions may be managed differently from those with multiple adenomatous polyposis. Although there may be more than one type of histopathological finding present, the predominant subtype should be adenomatous.

Classic FAP

Classic FAP may be characterized by hundreds to thousands of adenomatous colorectal polyps and accounts for less than 1% of all colorectal cancers.[2] Although most patients with FAP have a family history of the condition, up to 25% represent the first-recognized mutation in the family.[3] These patients are likely to have colorectal cancer at the time of presentation. The median age for adenoma development in patients with FAP is 17 years. Untreated patients develop colorectal cancer at a median age of 40 years, and death occurs by age 44 years.[2] In patients with FAP, an upper endoscopy may reveal gastric fundic gland polyps and gastric and duodenal adenomas. Extraintestinal manifestations of FAP on history or physical examination may include congenital hypertrophy of the retinal pigment epithelium (CHRPE), osteomas, fibromas, lipomas, epidermoid cysts, supernumerary teeth, and desmoid tumors. Other cancers such as medulloma, papillary thyroid cancer, or pediatric hepatoblastoma may also be associated with FAP.[4–6]

AFAP

Patients with AFAP may have between 1 and 100 adenomatous polyps (usually<50), and the polyps tend to be smaller and flatter.[7] As in classic FAP, there can be a wide variation in the number of polyps between members of the same kindred. The distribution of polyps tends to be more right sided, and rectal sparing is more likely. Polyps and colorectal cancer occur later than in classic FAP, at mean ages of 44 and 56 years, respectively.[7] Patients with AFAP may have gastric fundic gland polyps, gastric or duodenal adenomas, and periampullary tumors. CHRPE, osteomas, and desmoids are rarely reported in patients with AFAP.[7]

Lynch Syndrome

Lynch syndrome is more common than FAP and accounts for 2% to 3% of all colorectal cancers.[8,9] Patients who meet the Amsterdam Criteria (**Box 1**) and have an MMR mutation are referred to as having the Lynch syndrome. Those patients who

> **Box 1**
> **Amsterdam II Criteria**
>
> At least 3 relatives who have a hereditary nonpolyposis colorectal cancer (HNPCC)-associated cancer (colorectal, endometrial, ureter, renal pelvis, small bowel)
>
> One is a first-degree relative of the other two
>
> At least 2 generations are affected
>
> At least 1 relative was diagnosed at 50 years of age or earlier
>
> FAP has been excluded
>
> *Data from* Vasen HF, Mecklin JP, Khan PM, et al. The International Collaborative Group on Hereditary Non-Polyposis Colorectal Cancer (ICG-HNPCC). Dis Colon Rectum 1991;34(5):424–5.

meet the Amsterdam Criteria but do not have an MMR mutation are referred to as having FCC X.[10,11]

The phenotype of a patient with Lynch syndrome may include multiple adenomatous polyps and early age of onset of colorectal, endometrial, and other cancers. Colorectal cancer occurs at an average age of 45 years, and the adenoma to carcinoma sequence may be accelerated.[12] The history may reveal multiple HNPCC-associated cancers in the individual or family. Colorectal cancers tend to be right sided in Lynch syndrome, in contrast to the sporadic colorectal cancer, which shows a left-sided predominance. Histologic evaluation of the adenoma or cancer may show lymphocytic infiltration. Cancers are more likely to be poorly differentiated, heterogeneous, and of the medullary, mucinous, or signet-ring cell types.[13]

FCC X

Patients with FCC X may appear similar to patients with Lynch syndrome because their family history meets the Amsterdam Criteria. However, the major distinguishing feature of patients with FCC X from those with Lynch syndrome is the absence of a detectable MMR mutation. In addition, those with FCC X are more likely to have left-sided cancer and present at a slightly older age (55 vs 41 years).[14] Overall, FCC X tumors tend to be better differentiated, more often aneuploid, and less mucinous compared with the microsatellite unstable tumors in Lynch syndrome.[15]

MAP

Estimations of the prevalence of MAP are from 26% to 50% in patients with 10 to 100 adenomatous polyps and 7% to 29% in patients with 100 to 1000 polyps.[16] Adenomas or colorectal cancers tend to be detected between the fourth and seventh decade of life.[17] However, because MAP has an autosomal recessive pattern of inheritance with variable penetrance, the family history is more likely to be negative or subtle compared with that for the autosomal dominant syndromes. In some studies, the extraintestinal manifestations of this syndrome are not clearly defined but appear to include an increased risk of duodenal polyposis; ovarian, bladder, and sebaceous skin cancers; and an increased risk of breast cancer.[17,18] Gastric adenomas and fundic gland polyps have also been described. There are no pathologic features specifically associated with MAP polyps or cancers. However, cancers have been disproportionately found in the proximal colon.[19]

Because family history may not be well known and extracolonic manifestations may not be evident, genetic testing is often required in patients with multiple adenomatous polyps.

GENETIC TESTING

An important component of genetic testing is both pre- and posttest genetic counseling. Unfortunately, this testing is not always performed.[20] Genetic testing begins with a family member who is known to express the phenotype of the syndrome being tested to establish that the test will be informative in the family. The phenotype and clinical presentation can guide the testing for polyposis syndromes. A family history of extensive polyposis transmitted in an autosomal dominant fashion may suggest testing for an APC mutation first, whereas a family history of multiple early-age-of-onset colorectal and other cancers may suggest testing for Lynch syndrome initially. It has been suggested by some investigators that patients with more than 10 to 20 adenomatous polyps should be considered for APC and MUTYH mutation testing.[21,22] APC and MUTYH testing use the DNA obtained from peripheral leukocytes for gene sequencing.

When the phenotype and history suggest Lynch syndrome and cancer tissue is available, testing may begin with immunohistochemical (IHC) staining for the loss of MMR proteins.[11] The MMR genes, *MLH1*, *MSH2*, *MSH6*, and *PMS2*, code for proteins that repair base mismatches in DNA. IHC staining uses antibodies to the MMR proteins produced by the MMR genes. A lack of staining for a particular protein indicates a possible mutation of that gene. Although the sensitivity and specificity of IHC testing is excellent when performed on cancer tissue, only 70% of adenomas have an abnormal IHC in patients with a known MMR mutation.[23,24]

An alternative and equally effective option to IHC testing is microsatellite instability (MSI) testing.[25] MSI refers to the expansion or contraction of areas of DNA that are composed of short repeating sequences of nucleotides. MSI testing compares the length of microsatellites in tumor DNA to that in normal DNA from blood or normal tissue. The Bethesda Guidelines (**Box 2**) were established to determine which patients with colorectal cancer should undergo MSI testing. However, only 58% of adenomatous polyps demonstrate MSI in patients with known MMR mutations.[23] Because the yield for MSI and IHC testing is lower in adenomatous polyps than in cancer, gene sequencing should be performed on the patient who presents with multiple adenomatous polyps when Lynch syndrome is suspected. If the involved gene is known from another affected family member or based on the loss of a specific MMR protein detected on IHC testing, only that gene needs to be sequenced. Otherwise, the entire gene may need to be sequenced unless the patient is from a family that meets the Amsterdam Criteria and is of Ashkenazi Jewish descent, in which case rapid

---

Box 2
Revised Bethesda Guidelines for the testing of colorectal tumors for MSI

Individuals who meet any of the following criteria:

Colorectal cancer diagnosed at 50 years of age or earlier

Two HNPCC-related cancers (synchronous or metachronous)

Colorectal cancer with MSI-high histology at 60 years of age or earlier

First-degree relative who has HNPCC-related cancer, one of the cancers diagnosed at 50 years of age or earlier

Colorectal cancer in 2 or more first- or second-degree relatives with HNPCC-related tumors

Data from Umar A, Boland CR, Terdiman JP, et al. Revised Bethesda Guidelines for hereditary nonpolyposis colorectal cancer (Lynch syndrome) and microsatellite instability. J Natl Cancer Inst 2004;96(4):261–8.

single-amplicon testing for a specific mutation in the *MSH2* gene may be pursued.[26] When a tumor does not show loss of MMR proteins on IHC testing or is MSI stable and there are multiple polyps present, testing for MUTYH or APC mutations may be pursued.

Approximately 40% of patients meeting the Amsterdam Criteria may test negative for genetic abnormalities in the MMR genes.[27] These patients fall into the category of FCC X. In these cases, it is difficult to assess patients' risk of extraintestinal manifestations. The largest study to date found no statistically increased risk for other cancers.[10] However, other studies have shown a potential for association with a variety of other tumors.[17]

MAP is caused by variants in the base excision repair gene, MUTYH. In North America, the carrier frequency has been reported to be 2%.[28] MAP represents the only known colorectal cancer syndrome with autosomal recessive inheritance; this inheritance pattern can make a family colorectal cancer history more difficult to detect. For example, parents and offspring of the proband patient may not be affected, whereas siblings of the proband have a 25% chance of carrying biallelic mutations. Testing the other unaffected parent helps to assess if the children are at risk. Testing for MUTYH mutations may be done when the result of APC testing is negative; some laboratories test for both APC and MUTYH mutations simultaneously.

Some patients present with multiple adenomatous polyps but without a family history suggestive of a colorectal cancer syndrome and test negative for a known genetic mutation. These patients may harbor a de novo mutation, may be a member of a not-yet-identified kindred, or may harbor a mutation that is not detected by currently available testing technology. If the results of a clinical genetic workup are negative, patients can be counseled that the potential for an underlying inherited predisposition to developing colorectal cancer cannot be ruled out and that they should continue to undergo close surveillance if the colon can be cleared of polyps. If colonoscopic polypectomy cannot clear the colon, the patient should be offered a prophylactic colectomy.

SURVEILLANCE

If surgery is not indicated or desired at the time of the initial evaluation, surveillance of the colon is critical in patients with adenomatous multiple polyps. Patients should be advised about the potential risk of developing colorectal cancer while under surveillance. The age to commence colonoscopic examination and the frequency are determined by the genetic syndrome and phenotype.

Patients with FAP may undergo colonoscopy on an annual basis, beginning at approximately 12 years of age or earlier, if symptoms are present.[29] Multiple biopsies may be obtained from adenomas throughout the colon, particularly of large adenomas. Patients with AFAP may undergo colonoscopies on an annual basis as well.

Patients with multiple adenomas and an MMR mutation may undergo colonoscopy every 1 to 2 years, beginning at age 20 to 25 years or at an age 10 years younger than the youngest age of colorectal cancer diagnosed in the family.[30] However, if the patient is found to have polyps that cannot be managed endoscopically, surgery may be indicated. A prospective trial demonstrated a 63% decrease in the risk of colorectal cancer in patients with Lynch syndrome who underwent colonoscopy at 3-year intervals.[31] A more recent study showed that 1- to 2-year intervals further decreased cancer risk and that cancers were more likely to be detected at an earlier stage with a more frequent regimen.[32]

Individuals with FCC X have a 2-fold risk of developing colorectal cancer compared with the general population but appear to be at a lower risk compared with patients with Lynch syndrome.[10] There are no specific guidelines for colonoscopic surveillance for patients with FCC X. Some investigators suggest a surveillance regimen customized by pedigree and colonoscopic findings.[10] The authors and some other investigators suggest using the guidelines for patients with Lynch syndrome in the population with FCC X.[33]

Some investigators suggest that colonoscopic surveillance for biallelic MUTYH carriers may commence by about age 18 to 20 years and the follow-up interval may be 2 to 3 years.[34,35] However, this suggestion is not based on any evidence specific to MAP; it is based on the overall lifetime risk and the average age of adenoma and cancer onset. In patients with multiple adenomatous polyps and no specific mutation detected or family history of mutation, regular screening may be individualized based on phenotype.

Polyposis syndromes have associated benign and malignant extracolonic manifestations. FAP is associated with an increased risk for papillary thyroid cancer, desmoid tumors, and duodenal or periampullary adenomas with a risk of carcinoma. Lynch syndrome is associated with the development of a variety of extracolonic cancers, including those of the small bowel, stomach, ureter, renal pelvis, pancreas, biliary tract, endometrium, ovaries, and brain. Some investigators have also suggested associations of the syndrome with breast and prostate cancers. The risks associated with MAP are not as well defined but may include duodenal polyposis; ovarian, bladder, and skin cancers; and possibly an increased risk of breast cancer.[17] Referral for appropriate screening is an important component of managing patients with these syndromes. Patient education is also important to ensure that they pursue appropriate follow-up.

MEDICAL TREATMENT

Although chemoprevention is not recommended as a primary treatment in patients with multiple adenomatous polyps, it may serve as an adjunct to treatment in some patients. The goal is to reduce the appearance of new polyps and possibly induce regression of existing ones. Chemoprevention may potentially delay the need for surgery and perhaps lengthen the time for which polyposis can be managed endoscopically. Sulindac has been shown to suppress the formation of adenomas and to induce the regression of existing adenomas in adult patients with FAP, resulting in a 35% to 44% decrease in polyp burden.[36] The selective cyclooxygenase-2 inhibitor celecoxib was also found to reduce colorectal adenomas up to 30% in adult patients with FAP.[37] Small studies suggest similar results in children.[38] Although celecoxib may cause adenoma regression, it does not seem to prevent adenomas from occurring.[39] In a large-scale trial of patients taking celecoxib with or without aspirin, 0.9% of patients experienced cardiovascular events when taking both drugs and 0.5% when taking celecoxib without aspirin. The risk of cardiovascular events in patients taking nonsteroidal antiinflammatory drugs (NSAIDs) with and without aspirin was 1.0% and 0.4%, respectively.[40] However, some investigators believe that the benefit of adenoma suppression may outweigh this risk in the population with FAP. NSAIDs have also been used postcolectomy with ileorectal anastomosis (IRA) to decrease rectal polyp burden. There seems to be a slight decrease in the number of polyps with 6 months of use.[36] However, some investigators have suggested the possibility that resistance to therapy may occur over time and that the early results are not durable.[41] Early data concerning the omega-3 polyunsaturated fatty acid eicosapentaenoic acid (EPA) in adult patients with FAP show that EPA may be associated with a decrease in the number and size of polyps after 6 months of use, making it a target for further research.[42] Patients still require careful surveillance while using these treatments.

Observational data indicate that aspirin reduces the risk of sporadic colon cancer.[43] The Concerted Action Polyp Prevention II trial studied chemoprevention in patients with Lynch syndrome. Aspirin and resistant starch, individually, both, or neither, were given to patients with MMR gene mutations who either did not have polyps or had polyps that had been removed endoscopically. This study found no difference in adenoma development or cancer between the groups.[44] Based on the results in sporadic adenomas, resistant starch at higher doses may be effective, but this is an area for investigation.[45] At present, there is no known effective chemoprevention for this group of patients.

SURGICAL TREATMENT
FAP and AFAP

Because less than 1% of patients with FAP are diagnosed with cancer before 20 years of age, prophylactic surgery is recommended to take place in the late teens or early 20s.[35,46] Polyp burden is also considered because it correlates with the risk for colorectal cancer. Patients with severe polyposis, severe dysplasia, tubulovillous histopathology, multiple adenomas larger than 5 mm, and symptoms related to polyps should undergo surgery as soon as it is practical.[47] Surgical options include colectomy with IRA, proctocolectomy with ileal pouch–anal anastomosis (IPAA), or total proctocolectomy with permanent ileostomy.

The number and size of rectal polyps help to determine whether it is safe to leave the rectum in place. Usually, if there are fewer than 20 adenomas, all smaller than 1 cm and none with dysplasia, IRA is considered reasonable.[48] The postoperative function after IRA is excellent. The long-term risk of developing cancer in the remaining rectum is estimated to be 4% at 5 years and 25% at 20 years.[49] The risk is significantly higher if there are more than 20 rectal adenomas or 1000 colonic adenomas at the time of surgery or if the APC mutation is at the 3' end of codon 1250, between codon 1250 and 1464, in codon 1309, or in codon 1328.[48,50–52] A study that divided patients into 3 genotypic groups predicting attenuated, intermediate, and severe polyposis based on the location of the mutation found that the cumulative risk of secondary proctectomy and rectal cancer increased with each of the groups as expected. However, even in the lowest-risk group, rectal cancers occurred and proctectomies were required.[53] Although the concept of using genotype-phenotype relations to help guide the management of a specific patient is appealing, it is important to recognize the variability of phenotypic expression for each genotype. At present, the choice of surgical procedure should be based primarily on clinical rather than genetic grounds. Overall, up to 40% of patients who have undergone IRA require completion proctectomy later because of diffuse polyposis, functional problems, or rectal cancer. However, this number is decreasing as patient selection for IRA has changed with time.[54]

The total proctocolectomy with IPAA completely removes the colon and rectum. Continence is reported to be excellent in many patients, but there is a higher risk of decreased control than in those who have undergone IRA.[55] The incidence of adenomas in the pouch is 42% at 7 years after pouch construction, with higher rates for double-stapled anastomoses than for hand-sewn anastamoses.[56] The cumulative risk of carcinoma in the pouch is approximately 1% at 10 years.[56] Lifetime surveillance of the rectal remnant after IRA or the pouch in IPAA is therefore required.

Occasionally, patients may require or elect for total proctocolectomy with ileostomy. Reasons for this may include poor baseline sphincter function, invasive cancer involving the sphincters, or inability to successfully complete IPAA because of anatomic limitations or desmoid disease. Some patients choose this procedure as the primary procedure because of the perception that their lifestyle may be compromised by the frequent bowel movements sometimes associated with the IPAA procedure.[27]

Both IRA and IPAA can be performed as either an open or laparoscopic procedure. When performed laparoscopically, these procedures usually have longer operative times, similar morbidity and reoperation rates, and decreased intraoperative blood loss compared with open surgery. The postoperative course of patients undergoing laparoscopic procedures is notable for earlier return of bowel function and resumption of diet and decreased or equivalent hospital stay. Postoperative pain and narcotic requirements are decreased.[57] With regard to long-term functional outcomes of IPAA, matched cohorts of patients with open and laparoscopic procedures have shown equivalent number of times of defecation per 24 hours and equal continence rates.[58] Studies of postoperative quality of life and cosmesis show no difference in long-term outcomes, regardless of open or laparoscopic procedure.[59]

A population-based study showed that fecundity was decreased in patients with FAP undergoing IPAA, although not to the same extent as in those with ulcerative colitis who had undergone IPAA; notably, fecundity was not decreased after IRA.[60] However, another study of women with FAP came to a different conclusion. In this study, there was no change in fertility based on the type of surgery (IRA, IPAA, or total proctocolectomy with ileostomy), indication, or complications. The only factors that affected fertility were the age at diagnosis and age at first surgical procedure.[61] Some investigators suggest that it may be worthwhile to consider IRA as the initial surgery in young women desiring children, with a plan for completion proctectomy and IPAA if indicated, at a later date.[60]

Desmoids are the second most common cause of death in patients with FAP, after colon cancer.[62] Desmoids occur in up to 17% of the population with FAP, tend to be intra-abdominal, and occur after abdominal surgery.[63–65] Although intra-abdominal desmoids are rare before surgery, if present, they can affect the ability to perform an IPAA.[66] Risk factors for desmoids that can be determined preoperatively include female gender, extracolonic manifestations of FAP, and a family history of desmoids.[67] In carefully selected asymptomatic patients with a family history of aggressive abdominal desmoid disease, delaying surgery may be considered. Some investigators suggest that young nulliparous women may benefit from delaying surgery, undergoing a laparoscopic procedure, and undergoing IRA instead of an IPAA when feasible to avoid desmoid occurrence.[67,68]

When there is carcinoma at presentation, the goal of the intervention changes to controlling the cancer. The appropriate surgical approach may be the one that allows the patient to proceed with an adjuvant therapy, if necessary, as quickly as possible. This approach may include a temporary stoma or an IRA. Later, the stoma can be reversed, and if indicated, the IRA can be converted to an IPAA.

AFAP can be highly variable. In very select patients with a very low polyp burden, there is potential for nonoperative management via regular endoscopic surveillance and polypectomy. With higher polyp burdens, the options are similar to those for patients with classic FAP. The attenuated phenotype with relative rectal sparing more frequently permits IRA.

Lynch Syndrome

Lynch syndrome is marked by variable penetrance. Unlike FAP, there is a lifetime risk of 80%, but not 100%, for colorectal cancer in affected patients.[27] Prophylactic surgery may be considered when the polyp burden cannot be managed endoscopically, when colonoscopy is technically difficult to complete, or if the patient is not willing to undergo regular follow-up. Theoretical models predict an increased life expectancy of 1 to 2 years if prophylactic colectomy is performed at 25 or 30 years of age.[69,70]

Many patients with Lynch syndrome have cancer at the time of surgery, altering the goals of intervention. Oncologic treatment and minimizing recurrence risks are the primary considerations. Surgical options may include segmental colectomy, subtotal colectomy and IRA, and proctosigmoidectomy or total proctocolectomy. Proctectomy and proctocolectomy are indicated when rectal cancer is present. The need for permanent ileostomy is determined by the involvement and preoperative function of the anal sphincter complex.

Because of the high rate of metachronous colorectal neoplasms in patients with Lynch syndrome, total colectomy rather than segmental colectomy is the recommended surgical procedure in a patient presenting with a colorectal cancer.[27] Total colectomy at initial operation has been reported to lead to fewer abdominal surgeries than segmental colectomy.[71] Despite these considerations, there are no trials to demonstrate an improvement in survival in patients undergoing a more extensive resection at the time of initial surgery. Segmental resection requires close periodic colonoscopy, whereas surveillance after subtotal colectomy requires only flexible sigmoidoscopy. This need for colonoscopy may affect quality of life in some patients.[71]

When a female patient with Lynch syndrome undergoes colon surgery, prophylactic hysterectomy and oophorectomy may be done at the same time because of the increased risk for gynecologic cancers in these patients.[72] This option may depend on the age of the patient and her desires regarding future childbearing.

FCC X

Surgical treatment should be based on the phenotype of the patient and patient preferences. Prophylactic surgery is recommended only when polyps cannot be managed endoscopically. There are no data about the risk of metachronous cancers, so it is not known if subtotal colectomy would offer any benefit over segmental colectomy at the time of surgery for cancer.

MAP

In many cases, adenomatous polyp burden is low and may be managed endoscopically.[16] Surgery is recommended when the polyps are not amenable to endoscopic management. At present, there is no consensus on prophylactic surgery for affected patients. Some investigators recommend endoscopic surveillance, whereas others believe that the high rate of carcinoma is an indication for preemptive surgery.[73,74] When cancer is diagnosed, the principles of surgical intervention are the same as those for other high-risk syndromes.

SUMMARY

Patients with multiple adenomatous polyps may be at high risk for colorectal cancer. A detailed clinical history, family history, and physical examination, combined with the results of diagnostic tests, may suggest a specific hereditary syndrome. Genetic counseling and testing should be recommended in appropriate cases. Although chemoprevention with NSAIDs may be used, colonoscopic surveillance and surgery are the mainstays of treatment for these patients. The extent and timing of surgical intervention for the patient with multiple adenomatous polyps vary depending on the syndrome and its phenotypic expression.

REFERENCES

1. Heitman S, Ronksley P, Hilsden R, et al. Prevalence of adenomas and colorectal cancer in average risk individuals: a systematic review and meta-analysis. Clin Gastroenterol Hepatol 2009;7(12):1272–8.
2. Bulow S. Results of national registration of familial adenomatous polyposis. Gut 2003;52(5):742–6.
3. Aretz S, Uhlhaas S, Caspari R, et al. Frequency and parental origin of de novo APC mutations in familial adenomatous polyposis. Eur J Hum Genet 2004;12(1):52–8.
4. Herraiz M, Barbesino G, Faquin W, et al. Prevalence of thyroid cancer in familial adenomatous polyposis syndrome and the role of screening ultrasound examinations. Clin Gastroenterol Hepatol 2007;5(3):367–73.
5. Hughes LJ, Michels VV. Risk of hepatoblastoma in familial adenomatous polyposis. Am J Med Genet 1992;43(6):1023–5.
6. Paraf F, Jothy S, Van Meir EG. Brain tumor-polyposis syndrome: two genetic diseases? J Clin Oncol 1997;15(7):2744–58.
7. Hernegger GS, Moore HG, Guillem JG. Attenuated familial adenomatous polyposis: an evolving and poorly understood entity. Dis Colon Rectum 2002;45(1): 127–34 [discussion: 134–6].
8. Salovaara R, Loukola A, Kristo P, et al. Population-based molecular detection of hereditary nonpolyposis colorectal cancer. J Clin Oncol 2000;18(11):2193–200.
9. Cunningham JM, Kim CY, Christensen ER, et al. The frequency of hereditary defective mismatch repair in a prospective series of unselected colorectal carcinomas. Am J Hum Genet 2001;69(4):780–90.
10. Lindor N, Rabe K, Petersen G, et al. Lower cancer incidence in Amsterdam-I Criteria families without mismatch repair deficiency: familial colorectal cancer type X. JAMA 2005;293(16):1979–85.
11. Umar A, Boland CR, Terdiman JP, et al. Revised Bethesda Guidelines for hereditary nonpolyposis colorectal cancer (Lynch syndrome) and microsatellite instability. J Natl Cancer Inst 2004;96(4):261–8.
12. Jass JR. Pathology of hereditary nonpolyposis colorectal cancer. Ann N Y Acad Sci 2000;910:62–73 [discussion: 73–4].
13. Shia J, Ellis N, Paty P, et al. Value of histopathology in predicting microsatellite instability in hereditary nonpolyposis colorectal cancer and sporadic colorectal cancer. Am J Surg Pathol 2003;27(11):1407–17.
14. Mueller-Koch Y, Vogelsang H, Kopp R, et al. Hereditary non-polyposis colorectal cancer: clinical and molecular evidence for a new entity of hereditary colorectal cancer. Gut 2005;54(12):1733–40.
15. Valle L, Perea J, Carbonell P, et al. Clinicopathologic and pedigree differences in Amsterdam I-positive hereditary nonpolyposis colorectal cancer families according to tumor microsatellite instability status. J Clin Oncol 2007;25(7):781–6.
16. Nielsen M, Joerink-van de Beld MC, Jones N, et al. Analysis of MUTYH genotypes and colorectal phenotypes in patients With MUTYH-associated polyposis. Gastroenterology 2009;136(2):471–6.
17. Vogt S, Jones N, Christian D, et al. Expanded extracolonic tumor spectrum in MUTYH-associated polyposis. Gastroenterology 2009;137(6):1976–85, e1–10.
18. Lynch HT, Lynch JF, Attard TA. Diagnosis and management of hereditary colorectal cancer syndromes: Lynch syndrome as a model. CMAJ 2009;181(5):273–80.
19. Cleary SP, Cotterchio M, Jenkins MA, et al. Germline MutY human homologue mutations and colorectal cancer: a multisite case-control study. Gastroenterology 2009;136(4):1251–60.

20. Giardiello FM, Brensinger JD, Petersen GM, et al. The use and interpretation of commercial APC gene testing for familial adenomatous polyposis. N Engl J Med 1997;336(12):823–7.
21. Hampel H. Genetic testing for hereditary colorectal cancer. Surg Oncol Clin N Am 2009;18(4):687–703.
22. Giardiello FM, Brensinger JD, Petersen GM. AGA technical review on hereditary colorectal cancer and genetic testing. Gastroenterology 2001;121(1):198–213.
23. Pino M, Mino-Kenudson M, Wildemore B, et al. Deficient DNA mismatch repair is common in Lynch syndrome-associated colorectal adenomas. J Mol Diagn 2009; 11(3):238–47.
24. Evaluation of Genomic Applications in Practice and Prevention (EGAPP) Working Group. Recommendations from the EGAPP Working Group: genetic testing strategies in newly diagnosed individuals with colorectal cancer aimed at reducing morbidity and mortality from Lynch syndrome in relatives. Genet Med 2009;11(1):35–41.
25. Baudhuin LM, Burgart LJ, Leontovich O, et al. Use of microsatellite instability and immunohistochemistry testing for the identification of individuals at risk for lynch syndrome. Fam Cancer 2005;4(3):255–65.
26. Guillem JG, Glogowski E, Moore HG, et al. Single-amplicon MSH2 A636P mutation testing in Ashkenazi Jewish patients with colorectal cancer: role in presurgical management. Ann Surg 2007;245(4):560–5.
27. Guillem J, Wood W, Moley J, et al. ASCO/SSO review of current role of risk-reducing surgery in common hereditary cancer syndromes. J Clin Oncol 2006; 24(28):4642–60.
28. Croitoru ME, Cleary SP, Di Nicola N, et al. Association between biallelic and monoallelic germline MYH gene mutations and colorectal cancer risk. J Natl Cancer Inst 2004;96(21):1631–4.
29. Levin B, Lieberman D, McFarland B, et al. Screening and surveillance for the early detection of colorectal cancer and adenomatous polyps, 2008: a joint guideline from the American Cancer Society, the US Multi-Society Task Force on Colorectal Cancer, and the American College of Radiology. CA Cancer J Clin 2008;58(3):130–60.
30. Lindor NM, Petersen GM, Hadley DW, et al. Recommendations for the care of individuals with an inherited predisposition to Lynch syndrome: a systematic review. JAMA 2006;296(12):1507–17.
31. Jarvinen HJ, Aarnio M, Mustonen H, et al. Controlled 15-year trial on screening for colorectal cancer in families with hereditary nonpolyposis colorectal cancer. Gastroenterology 2000;118(5):829–34.
32. Vasen HFA, Abdirahman M, Brohet R, et al. One to 2-year surveillance intervals reduce risk of colorectal cancer in families with Lynch syndrome. Gastroenterology 2010;138(7):2300–6.
33. Rex D, Johnson D, Anderson J, et al. American College of Gastroenterology guidelines for colorectal cancer screening 2009 [corrected]. Am J Gastroenterol 2009;104(3):739–50.
34. Lubbe S, Di Bernardo M, Chandler I, et al. Clinical implications of the colorectal cancer risk associated with *MUTYH* mutation. J Clin Oncol 2009;27(24):3975–80.
35. Vasen HF, Moslein G, Alonso A, et al. Guidelines for the clinical management of familial adenomatous polyposis (FAP). Gut 2008;57(5):704–13.
36. Giardiello FM, Hamilton SR, Krush AJ, et al. Treatment of colonic and rectal adenomas with sulindac in familial adenomatous polyposis. N Engl J Med 1993;328(18):1313–6.

37. Steinbach G, Lynch PM, Phillips RK, et al. The effect of celecoxib, a cyclooxyge-nase-2 inhibitor, in familial adenomatous polyposis. N Engl J Med 2000;342(26): 1946–52.
38. Lynch P, Ayers G, Hawk E, et al. The safety and efficacy of celecoxib in children with familial adenomatous polyposis. Am J Gastroenterol 2010;105(6):1437–43.
39. Giardiello FM, Yang VW, Hylind LM, et al. Primary chemoprevention of familial adenomatous polyposis with sulindac. N Engl J Med 2002;346(14):1054–9.
40. Silverstein FE, Faich G, Goldstein JL, et al. Gastrointestinal toxicity with celecoxib vs nonsteroidal anti-inflammatory drugs for osteoarthritis and rheumatoid arthritis: the CLASS study: a randomized controlled trial. Celecoxib Long-term Arthritis Safety Study. JAMA 2000;284(10):1247–55.
41. Cruz-Correa M, Hylind LM, Romans KE, et al. Long-term treatment with sulindac in familial adenomatous polyposis: a prospective cohort study. Gastroenterology 2002;122(3):641–5.
42. West N, Clark S, Phillips RKS, et al. Eicosapentaenoic acid reduces rectal polyp number and size in familial adenomatous polyposis. Gut 2010;59(7): 918–25.
43. Baron JA, Cole BF, Sandler RS, et al. A randomized trial of aspirin to prevent colo-rectal adenomas. N Engl J Med 2003;348(10):891–9.
44. Burn J, Bishop DT, Mecklin J-P, et al. Effect of aspirin or resistant starch on colo-rectal neoplasia in the Lynch syndrome. N Engl J Med 2008;359(24):2567–78.
45. Yang F, Jin C, Fu D. Effect of aspirin or resistant starch on colorectal neoplasia in the Lynch syndrome. N Engl J Med 2009;360(14):1461–2.
46. Jasperson K, Tuohy T, Neklason D, et al. Hereditary and familial colon cancer. Gastroenterology 2010;138(6):2044–58.
47. Church J, Simmang C. Practice parameters for the treatment of patients with dominantly inherited colorectal cancer (familial adenomatous polyposis and hereditary nonpolyposis colorectal cancer). Dis Colon Rectum 2003;46(8): 1001–12.
48. Church J, Burke C, McGannon E, et al. Risk of rectal cancer in patients after co-lectomy and ileorectal anastomosis for familial adenomatous polyposis: a function of available surgical options. Dis Colon Rectum 2003;46(9):1175–81.
49. Heiskanen I Jr, Vinen HJ. Fate of the rectal stump after colectomy and ileorectal anastomosis for familial adenomatous polyposis. Int J Colorectal Dis 1997;12(1): 9–13.
50. Wu JS, Paul P, McGannon EA, et al. APC genotype, polyp number, and surgical options in familial adenomatous polyposis. Ann Surg 1998;227(1):57–62.
51. Vasen HF, van der Luijt RB, Tops C, et al. Molecular genetic tests in surgical management of familial adenomatous polyposis. Lancet 1998;351(9109):1131–2.
52. Bertario L, Russo A, Radice P, et al. Genotype and phenotype factors as determi-nants for rectal stump cancer in patients with familial adenomatous polyposis. Hereditary colorectal tumors registry. Ann Surg 2000;231(4):538–43.
53. Nieuwenhuis M, Blow S, Bjrk J, et al. Genotype predicting phenotype in familial adenomatous polyposis: a practical application to the choice of surgery. Dis Colon Rectum 2009;52(7):1259–63.
54. Bulow S, Bulow C, Vasen H, et al. Colectomy and ileorectal anastomosis is still an option for selected patients with familial adenomatous polyposis. Dis Colon Rectum 2008;51(9):1318–23.
55. Aziz O, Athanasiou T, Fazio VW, et al. Meta-analysis of observational studies of ileorectal versus ileal pouch-anal anastomosis for familial adenomatous poly-posis. Br J Surg 2006;93(4):407–17.

56. Friederich P, de Jong A, Mathus-Vliegen L, et al. Risk of developing adenomas and carcinomas in the ileal pouch in patients with familial adenomatous polyposis. Clin Gastroenterol Hepatol 2008;6(11):1237–42.
57. Larson D, Cima R, Dozois E, et al. Safety, feasibility, and short-term outcomes of laparoscopic ileal-pouch-anal anastomosis: a single institutional case-matched experience. Ann Surg 2006;243(5):667–70.
58. El-Gazzaz GS, Kiran RP, Remzi FH, et al. Outcomes for case-matched laparoscopically assisted versus open restorative proctocolectomy. Br J Surg 2009; 96(5):522–6.
59. Larson D, Davies M, Dozois E, et al. Sexual function, body image, and quality of life after laparoscopic and open ileal pouch-anal anastomosis. Dis Colon Rectum 2008;51(4):392–6.
60. Olsen KO, Juul S, Bulow S, et al. Female fecundity before and after operation for familial adenomatous polyposis. Br J Surg 2003;90(2):227–31.
61. Nieuwenhuis MH, Douma KF, Bleiker EM, et al. Female fertility after colorectal surgery for familial adenomatous polyposis: a nationwide cross-sectional study. Ann Surg 2010;252(2):341–4.
62. Arvanitis ML, Jagelman DG, Fazio VW, et al. Mortality in patients with familial adenomatous polyposis. Dis Colon Rectum 1990;33(8):639–42.
63. Clark SK, Neale KF, Landgrebe JC, et al. Desmoid tumours complicating familial adenomatous polyposis. Br J Surg 1999;86(9):1185–9.
64. Soravia C, Berk T, McLeod RS, et al. Desmoid disease in patients with familial adenomatous polyposis. Dis Colon Rectum 2000;43(3):363–9.
65. Penna C, Tiret E, Parc R, et al. Operation and abdominal desmoid tumors in familial adenomatous polyposis. Surg Gynecol Obstet 1993;177(3):263–8.
66. Hartley JE, Church JM, Gupta S, et al. Significance of incidental desmoids identified during surgery for familial adenomatous polyposis. Dis Colon Rectum 2004; 47(3):334–8.
67. Elayi E, Manilich E, Church J. Polishing the crystal ball: knowing genotype improves ability to predict desmoid disease in patients with familial adenomatous polyposis. Dis Colon Rectum 2009;52(10):1762–6.
68. Heiskanen I, Jarvinen HJ. Occurrence of desmoid tumours in familial adenomatous polyposis and results of treatment. Int J Colorectal Dis 1996;11(4):157–62.
69. Syngal S, Weeks JC, Schrag D, et al. Benefits of colonoscopic surveillance and prophylactic colectomy in patients with hereditary nonpolyposis colorectal cancer mutations. Ann Intern Med 1998;129(10):787–96.
70. Vasen HF, Wijnen JT, Menko FH, et al. Cancer risk in families with hereditary non-polyposis colorectal cancer diagnosed by mutation analysis. Gastroenterology 1996;110(4):1020–7.
71. Natarajan N, Watson P, Silva-Lopez E, et al. Comparison of extended colectomy and limited resection in patients with Lynch syndrome. Dis Colon Rectum 2010; 53(1):77–82.
72. Boilesen AEB, Bisgaard M, Bernstein I. Risk of gynecologic cancers in Danish hereditary non-polyposis colorectal cancer families. Acta Obstet Gynecol Scand 2008;87(11):1129–35.
73. Lefevre JH, Rodrigue CM, Mourra N, et al. Implication of MYH in colorectal polyposis. Ann Surg 2006;244(6):874–9 [discussion: 879–80].
74. Balaguer F, Castellvi-Bel S, Castells A, et al. Identification of MYH mutation carriers in colorectal cancer: a multicenter, case-control, population-based study. Clin Gastroenterol Hepatol 2007;5(3):379–87.

How to Manage the Patient with Early-Age-of-Onset (<50 years) Colorectal Cancer?

Jennifer Liang, MBChB, James Church, MBChB, FRACS*

KEYWORDS

• Colorectal cancer • Early age of onset • Genetic abnormalities
• Young patient

Colorectal cancer occurs because of an accumulation of genetic abnormalities in a line of colonocytes that are usually the result of many years of exposure to environmental carcinogens. The genetic abnormalities produce cells that are capable of escaping controls on growth, death, and differentiation, and these cells are able to travel from their site of origin and establish viable colonies in distant locations. For cancer to develop, the neoplastic cells must also overcome the defense mechanisms of the host, which often recognize them as foreign and try to destroy them. The timing of the appearance of colorectal cancer is therefore the result of a balance of tumor factors and patient factors.

Colorectal cancer does not arise de novo from normal epithelium. There is a polyp-cancer sequence, the histology of which depends on the underlying genetic changes in the epithelial cells. Widespread mucosal methylation produces a serrated polyp-carcinoma pathway, but an adenoma-carcinoma sequence is the most common way in which the effect of accumulating mutations is expressed. For sporadic cancers, the time between the appearance of an adenoma and the change into carcinoma is approximately 10 years.[1]

The median age at diagnosis for colorectal cancer in the United States is 70 years, reflecting the overall time it takes for carcinogenesis to occur.[2] A young age at diagnosis suggests rapid carcinogenesis and is rare; approximately 5% of patients with colorectal cancer are diagnosed at age less than 45 years. A younger age at diagnosis is rarer, with 0.1% of all colorectal cancers diagnosed at age less than 20 years, 1.1% between 20 and 34 years, and 3.8% between 35 and 44 years. A further 12.4% are diagnosed

Department of Colorectal Surgery, Digestive Diseases Institute, Cleveland Clinic Foundation, Desk A30, 9500 Euclid Avenue, Cleveland, OH, USA
* Corresponding author.
E-mail address: churchj@ccf.org

Surg Oncol Clin N Am 19 (2010) 725–731
doi:10.1016/j.soc.2010.07.007
1055-3207/10/$ – see front matter © 2010 Elsevier Inc. All rights reserved.

between 45 and 54 years.[2] The accelerated carcinogenesis in these young patients may be caused by one or more of several possible factors, including particularly powerful environmental carcinogens, a particularly weak host response, and the inheritance of a germline mutation in a key tumor suppressor gene. When a young patient presents with a colorectal cancer, consideration of all these possibilities is helpful.

BIOLOGY OF COLORECTAL CANCER IN YOUNG PATIENTS

Many articles describe groups of young patients with colorectal cancer. O'Connell and colleagues[3] performed a thorough literature search and reviewed 55 reports mostly defining young as less than 40 years of age. Some interesting facts emerged. Although there was no difference in the proportion of men or women affected, African Americans were overrepresented in the young cancer group. Almost a quarter of the patients had a family history of colorectal cancer (22.7%, compared with 28.8% in a study of patients between 30 and 70 years of age[4]), and a further 16% had other predisposing factors, such as inflammatory bowel disease, hereditary colorectal cancer syndromes, and a family history of primary cancers in other organs. Delay in diagnosis was common in patients with colorectal cancer diagnosed at age less than 40 years and averaged a little more than 6 months. Most cancers were left sided (67%), and 66% were Dukes stage C or Turnbull stage D. There was a high incidence of mucinous tumors (21%) and poorly differentiated tumors (27%). Resectability rate was 86%, and 5-year survival rates were 94% (Dukes A), 76.5% (Dukes B), 39% (Dukes C), and 6.8% (stage D).

In a different study, the same authors reviewed the Surveillance Epidemiology and End Result (SEER) national database and compared patients with colorectal cancer who were aged between 20 and 40 years at diagnosis with those aged between 60 and 80 years.[5] Again, young patients were more often African American (16.4% vs 9.0%) and had tumors that were of more advanced stage (stages III and IV, 56% vs 41%) and more often poorly differentiated (27.3% vs 17.2%). Despite this, 5-year survival for stages I and III were similar between the 2 age groups, whereas survival after resection of stage II and IV cancers was better in young patients. There were no family history data available in the SEER database. There are thus several features of colorectal cancer in young patients that potentially affect diagnosis, workup and management.

Advanced Stage at Diagnosis

One obvious reason for the advanced disease that characterizes colorectal cancer in young patients is delay in diagnosis. Unless there is a family history, these patients are not screened, so cancers are usually symptomatic at presentation. Even when symptoms occur, they may be initially misdiagnosed. Rectal bleeding, for example, is often put down to an anorectal cause. O'Connell and colleagues[3] reported an average delay in diagnosis of 6.2 months, the reasons for which included a delay in presentation on the part of the patient, limited access to care, and misdiagnosis on the part of the physician. Minimizing delay in diagnosis means not taking symptoms lightly. Outlet-type bleeding usually has an anal cause, but when no anal cause is obvious and the bleeding persists, colonoscopy is mandatory, regardless of the patient's age. Abdominal pain is not usually a presenting symptom of colorectal cancer, nor is change in bowel habit. However, symptom persistence and the lack of a convincing alternative explanation for the symptoms demand further investigation.

Family History

A family history is an important part of the evaluation of each and every patient. Historically, physicians perform badly in the proportion of patients queried,[6–8] and the overall sensitivity of a family history of colorectal cancer varies from 0.6 for first-degree relatives to 0.3 for second degree.[8] However, despite limited accuracy and compliance, family history is still the most easily obtainable risk factor for colorectal cancer; a thorough family history is essential. Each generation is asked for specifically, and lack of knowledge is not equated to a knowledgeable "No." Any abdominal cancers, colonic polyps, need for a stoma, and extra-abdominal cancers, such as those of the uterus, ovary, liver, and small intestine, are queried for. A cancer-prone family may not fit any of the commonly recognized syndromes but may be at high risk of colorectal cancer nonetheless. When the proband is young and has a colorectal cancer, a weakly positive family history[9] is viewed with suspicion and a strongly positive family history of colorectal cancer is a clear indication of an inherited syndrome. The absence of polyposis and presence of a right-sided tumor suggest Lynch syndrome (hereditary DNA mismatch repair deficiency). It is important to diagnose this syndrome for several reasons. Firstly, the best surgical option in a patient with Lynch syndrome and a cancer is colectomy and ileorectal anastomosis, which is to prevent metachronous cancers. Secondly, patients with Lynch syndrome are at risk for cancers of other organs, making surveillance a consideration and raising the possibility of prophylactic hysterectomy and oophorectomy. Thirdly, patients suspected of Lynch syndrome can be offered genetic testing, which would establish the diagnosis, allow focused surveillance depending on the gene carrying the mutation, and make genetic analysis available to at-risk relatives. Young patients with colorectal cancer benefit from a consultation with a genetic counselor, who can take an accurate family history and make recommendations for genetic testing.

Colorectal cancer arising at a young age is a risk factor for the family of the patient. Johns and Houlston[10] performed a meta-analysis of 27 case-control and cohort studies of colorectal cancer risk and found that a family history of 1 affected first-degree relative who was diagnosed before the age of 45 carries a 3.87-fold (95% CI, 2.40–6.22) increased risk for the disease. Colonoscopic surveillance is recommended starting 10 years before the age of the youngest affected relative and is continued at 5-year intervals, or sooner if a polyp is found.

Other Predisposing Factors

Obvious factors such as chronic colitis and familial polyposis are relatively easily identified, and the patients may be managed by surveillance or prophylactic colectomy. MYH-associated polyposis (MAP), however, is sometimes not clinically obvious. This syndrome of mild or attenuated polyposis is recessively inherited, and therefore, family history may be weak or absent. The number of synchronous adenomas or serrated polyps[11] may be few, and so the syndrome may go undiagnosed. A proportion of young patients with colorectal cancer have MAP.[12] The tumors are microsatellite stable. Genetic testing should be considered.

Deficiencies in host response to carcinogenesis are less-easily recognized and less-easily treated. A personal history of other cancers, especially immunosensitive cancers such as melanoma, if occurring at a young age, may indicate an increased susceptibility to colorectal cancer. Chronic immune suppression or clinical suggestions of impaired immunity may also mean the same.

Advanced Biology

The advanced stage at presentation of many colorectal cancers in young patients is not just a result of a delay in diagnosis. The high proportion of mucinous and signet ring cell cancers suggests a disproportionate number of methylator tumors in this group.[13] The poor differentiation is typical of mutator tumors.[13] There are no data to support these conclusions, but such data are important, as they may influence the use of chemotherapy in the high proportion of cancers that have metastasized. The paradoxical good survival for patients with young age at diagnosis of colorectal cancer supports the idea that many cancers are microsatellite unstable, as this is the most common scenario in which survival after colon cancer resection is better than expected for grade and stage. However, crude survival is expected to be better than usual in young patients because of their youth and the improved tolerance of surgery and complications that this youth confers.

THE APPROACH TO THE YOUNG PATIENT WITH COLORECTAL CANCER

The approach to young patients with a colorectal cancer starts with the colonoscopy by which the diagnosis was made. If the diagnosis was made some other way, a colonoscopy is scheduled to exclude inflammatory bowel disease or polyposis and to biopsy the cancer. Biopsies are tested by standard hematoxylin-and-eosin light microscopy, as histologic features such as the presence of tumor infiltrating lymphocytes, a Crohn-type reaction, mucinous differentiation, and signet ring cells are suggestive of a tumor with defective DNA mismatch repair.[14] Tumor biopsies are tested for microsatellite instability. If the tumor is microsatellite unstable (MSI-H) and the family history is positive, Lynch syndrome is likely, and testing for a germline mutation should be requested. Alternatively, the biopsies can be tested by immunohistochemistry for the presence of DNA mismatch repair proteins. Absence of MSH2, PMS2, or MSH6 means Lynch syndrome and identifies the gene to be tested for a germline mutation. Absence of MLH1 may mean sporadic mismatch repair deficiency caused by promoter methylation, but with a positive family history, Lynch syndrome is more likely.

Colonoscopy also reveals the presence of synchronous polyps. More than 5 adenomas or serrated polyps is suggestive of the presence of a syndrome, either MAP or hyperplastic polyposis. If the tumor biopsy is microsatellite stable, genetic testing for MYH mutations should be sought, regardless of family history and associated adenomas.

At the time of colonoscopy, a detailed family history is taken. However, the family history is negative in about 22% of patients with familial adenomatous polyposis, may be negative or weak in patients with MAP, and may be falsely negative in patients with Lynch syndrome. If positive, family history is helpful. If negative, hereditary colorectal cancer is not necessarily ruled out. In such cases, genetic counseling is helpful and allows an appropriate risk calculation.

While the genetics of the cancer are being established, clinical staging is performed. The knowledge that colorectal cancers in young patients are more often advanced than those in older patients means that staging with a positron emission tomogram–enhanced CT scan is indicated. Tumor spread outside the scope of a standard segmental oncologic colectomy should be detected if possible and plans made to extend the colectomy or use adjuvant therapy to deal with the metastases. Because the patient is young, there is an inevitable tendency to be unusually aggressive in trying to cure a sometimes incurable situation. Accurate preoperative assessment is key to avoiding futile attempts at radical resections that lead to unnecessary morbidity.

For a stage I, II, or III cancer, a radical segmental colectomy is performed. If there is evidence of a hereditary syndrome in the patient's cancer (microsatellite instability, histologic signs as listed earlier, absent expression of a mismatch repair protein) or family history, a total or subtotal colectomy is recommended. This procedure minimizes the risk of a metachronous cancer and eases the dependence on faithful, accurate, yearly colonoscopy.[15] Postoperative adjuvant chemotherapy is indicated for node-positive disease and possibly for stage II disease with poor prognostic features (<12 nodes sampled, poor differentiation). Genetic characterization of the tumor (KRAS status, microsatellite status, gene expression array) is important for adjusting chemotherapy and may allow a more accurate identification of tumors at high risk for recurrence.

Follow-up includes colonoscopy at 1 year after surgery and then regularly every 2 to 3 years, depending on the signs of mucosal instability in the colon and the results of genetic testing that may have been performed. Multiple synchronous neoplasms are an indication for more frequent surveillance, whereas a solitary index lesion allows more relaxed scheduling. A history of predisposing factors or a suggestive family history demands yearly endoscopic surveillance. A hereditary cancer syndrome is

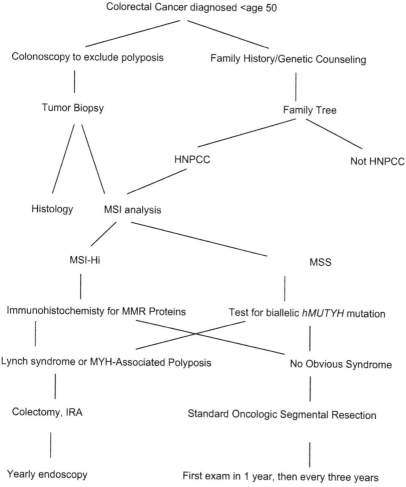

Fig. 1. An algorithmic approach to the management of young patients with colorectal cancer. HNPCC, hereditary nonpolyposis colorectal cancer; IRA, ileorectal anastomosis; MMR, mismatch repair; MSI, microsatellite instability; MSS, *microsatellite* stable.

an indication for regular surveillance of other organs. If Lynch syndrome is suspected or confirmed, prophylactic hysterectomy can be offered. The alternative is yearly pelvic ultrasonography after age 30 years, with biopsy of an abnormally thick endometrium. Esophagogastroduodenoscopy (EGD) is done at diagnosis as a baseline and then repeated every 3 to 5 years depending on the unfolding natural history of the patients' gastrointestinal tract. Urine cytology for transitional cell cancer has been suggested, but its usefulness has not been proven. A diagnosis of *familial adenomatous polyposis* or MAP requires regular EGD and thyroid ultrasound examinations. MAP may be associated with a high risk of renal cancer.

The patient's family is alerted, through the patient, of their increased risk for colorectal cancer. Depending on the results of family history and genetic testing of blood and tumor, genetic counseling and testing may be offered to the family. This approach is summarized in **Fig. 1.**

SUMMARY

Colorectal cancer rarely occurs before age 50 years. When it does, it is often advanced and aggressive. There may be predisposing genetic and immune factors that lead to its origin. Genetic counseling is indicated for all patients younger than 50 years with colorectal cancer. Before surgery, the tumor and the patient must be evaluated as fully as possible, so that optimal treatment, follow-up and surveillance are used.

REFERENCES

1. Winawer SJ, Zauber AG, Ho MN, et al. Prevention of colorectal cancer by colonoscopic polypectomy. The National Polyp Study Workgroup. N Engl J Med 1993; 329(27):1977–81.
2. Surveillance, Epidemiology, and End Results (SEER) Program. SEER*Stat Database: Incidence - SEER 11 Regs Public-Use, Nov 2001 Sub (1992–1999). Available at: http://www.seer.cancer.gov. Accessed July 31, 2010.
3. O'Connell JB, Maggard MA, Livingston EH, et al. Colorectal cancer in the young. Am J Surg 2004;187:343–8.
4. Mitchell RJ, Campbell H, Farrington SM, et al. Prevalence of family history of colorectal cancer in the general population. Br J Surg 2005;92(9):1161–4.
5. O'Connell JB, Maggard MA, Liu JH, et al. Do young colon cancer patients have worse outcomes? World J Surg 2004;28:558–62.
6. Murff HJ, Greevy RA, Syngal S. The comprehensiveness of family cancer history assessments in primary care. Community Genet 2007;10(3):174–80.
7. Church J, McGannon E. Family history of colorectal cancer: how often and how accurately is it recorded? Dis Colon Rectum 2000;43(11):1540–4.
8. Mitchell RJ, Brewster D, Campbell H, et al. Accuracy of reporting of family history of colorectal cancer. Gut 2004;53(2):291–5.
9. Church JM. A scoring system for the strength of a family history of colorectal cancer. Dis Colon Rectum 2005;48(5):889–96.
10. Johns LE, Houlston RS. A systematic review and meta-analysis of familial colorectal cancer risk. Am J Gastroenterol 2001;96(10):2992–3003.
11. Boparai KS, Dekker E, Van Eeden S, et al. Hyperplastic polyps and sessile serrated adenomas as a phenotypic expression of MYH-associated polyposis. Gastroenterology 2008;135(6):2014–8.
12. Balaguer F, Castellví-Bel S, Castells A, et al. Identification of MYH mutation carriers in colorectal cancer: a multicenter, case-control, population-based study. Clin Gastroenterol Hepatol 2007;5(3):379–87.

13. Sanchez JA, Krumroy L, Plummer S, et al. Genetic and epigenetic classifications define clinical phenotypes and determine patient outcomes in colorectal cancer. Br J Surg 2009;96(10):1196–204.
14. Greenson JK, Huang SC, Herron C, et al. Pathologic predictors of microsatellite instability in colorectal cancer. Am J Surg Pathol 2009;33(1):126–33.
15. Natarajan N, Watson P, Silva-Lopez E, et al. Comparison of extended colectomy and limited resection in patients with Lynch syndrome. Dis Colon Rectum 2010; 53(1):77–82.

Pretherapy Imaging of Rectal Cancers: ERUS or MRI?

Geerard L. Beets, MD, PhD[a,c],*, Regina G.H. Beets-Tan, MD, PhD[b,c]

KEYWORDS

- Endorectal ultrasonography • Rectal cancer • MRI
- Pretherapy imaging

Surgical treatment of rectal cancer has been plagued by a high local recurrence rate, until in the last decades the role of a good surgical technique and adjuvant (chemo)radiation was fully appreciated.[1] Additionally it was shown that (chemo)radiation was more effective when given before rather than after the resection.[2] Whereas previously most decisions on whether or not to give adjuvant treatment were based on the risk assessment for recurrence through histologic evaluation of the tumor and the lymph nodes, the decisions on neoadjuvant treatment now have to be based mainly on risk assessment through imaging. Although modern CT techniques are improving and are to some extent able to provide information for locoregional staging, endorectal ultrasonography (ERUS) and MRI are considered as the 2 best locoregional staging methods for rectal cancer. When comparing ERUS with MRI, there are several issues that require consideration. In addition to the accuracy in predicting a certain risk factor for local recurrence, there is the treatment strategy that dictates what information will have a clinical consequence, and there are also issues of expertise, availability, and cost. Currently, there is also a trend to study alternative treatment options after a good response to treatment, such as a local excision, or even a nonoperative wait-and-see approach. It is clear that imaging will play an important role in the selection and follow-up of these patients. This new role of imaging to detect small volumes of residual disease in the bowel wall and lymph nodes, sometimes within fibrotic scar tissue, is beyond the scope of this article.

[a] Department of Surgery, Maastricht University Medical Centre, PO Box 5800, 6202 AZ Maastricht, The Netherlands
[b] Division of Abdominal Radiology, Department of Radiology, Maastricht University Medical Centre, PO Box 5800, 6202 AZ Maastricht, The Netherlands
[c] GROW, School for Oncology & Developmental Biology, Maastricht University, PO Box 616, 6200 MD Maastricht, The Netherlands
* Corresponding author. Department of Surgery, Maastricht University Medical Centre, PO Box 5800, 6202 AZ Maastricht, The Netherlands.
E-mail addresses: g.beets@mumc.nl; g.beets@me.com

Surg Oncol Clin N Am 19 (2010) 733–741
doi:10.1016/j.soc.2010.07.004
1055-3207/10/$ – see front matter © 2010 Elsevier Inc. All rights reserved.

RISK FACTORS FOR LOCAL RECURRENCE

In large databases, the risk factors associated with local recurrence are generally similar to the risk factors for distant recurrence: T stage, N stage, distance to the circumferential resection margin (CRM), perineural invasion, lymph and blood vessel invasion, and histologic grade.[3,4] Of these risk factors, the T and N stage are commonly used for (neo)adjuvant treatment decisions,[5] and recently the distance to the CRM in clinical settings where a short course of radiotherapy is a treatment option.[6] There is a long history of classifying colorectal cancers using the depth of penetration through the bowel wall and lymph node invasion, a system that has been developed through histologic analysis of the resection specimen. The classification system is highly reproducible through the use of cutoff points that are usually straightforward histologically, such as the distinction between a T2 and T3 tumor depending on ingrowth in the mesorectum or not. This does not always easily transfer to staging through imaging. All imaging methods are good in showing the bulk of the tumor, but will have difficulty in predicting the exact microscopic relation to a histologic interface in a tumor that comes very near to this interface. It is therefore unrealistic to expect 100% accuracy from imaging technology in predicting a histologic classification. Imaging could be helpful in predicting risks for recurrence in its own right with volume and size as prognostic variables. Given the increasing use of preoperative (chemo)radiation in rectal cancer, this should be a topic for further studies. Meanwhile, imaging will continue to try to predict the histologic risk factors.

Tumor Stage

Endorectal ultrasound has been used to assess tumor ingrowth into the bowel wall since the mid 1980s after the description and the results of the technique by Hildebrandt and colleagues[7] and Beynon and colleagues.[8] The different layers of the rectal wall can be seen as 3 hyperechoic and 2 hypoechoic bands, corresponding to the anatomic layers and the interfaces between them. A tumor is shown as a hypoechoic mass. A good overview of staging with ERUS, including the more practical aspects, is provided by Edelman and Weiser.[9] The accuracy of the T-stage assessment in the smaller series is generally about 80% to 90%. Most of the studies are summarized in recent review articles[9–11] and a meta-analysis comparing ERUS, CT, and MRI.[12] Harewood[11] noted in his review that the larger and more recent studies show lower accuracy rates, and the overall accuracy of 85% in the literature may be an overestimate. Rather than focusing on an overall accuracy estimate, it is more helpful to address specific questions. The overall agreement between uT-stage and pT-stage in the larger studies is 63% to 69%, with 12% to 15% understaging and 18% to 24% overstaging.[13–16] In these series, there is understaging uT1 in 6% to 24%, and in uT2 stage 16% to 30%. Overstaging in uT3 occurred in 20% to 28%. Some series address the specific question of distinguishing mucosal T0 lesions from T1 tumors, showing a risk of understaging with uT0 of only 5% to 17%.[15,17–19] It is generally considered that ERUS is good in imaging the smaller tumors (**Fig. 1**). For the large lesion, ERUS can identify ingrowth in surrounding structures that are within the field of view such as vagina, prostate, and seminal vesicles. The difficulties arise with tumors located high in the rectum and stenosing tumors, and the overall limited field of view provides insufficient anatomic information in many large T3 to 4 tumors, as described in the section on CRM, later in this article.

Bipat and colleagues[12] published an extensive meta-analysis in 2004 comparing ERUS, CT, and MRI, including a variety of MR techniques and coils. Overall, the performance of ERUS in T staging was a little better than MRI. In their methodology,

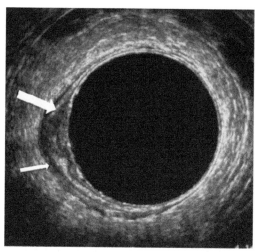

Fig. 1. ERUS showing a small tumor growing into the white hyperechoic layer that represents the submucosa (*large arrow*). It comes close to the dark hypoechoic layer that represents the muscular wall (*small arrow*), without obvious ingrowth. The tumor can therefore be classified as T1. (*Courtesy of* Dr Martin R. Weiser, New York, NY.)

the sensitivity and specificity of detecting muscularis propria invasion was 94% and 69% for MRI and 94% and 86% for ERUS. For the detection of perirectal tissue invasion, the sensitivity and specificity were 82% and 76% for MRI and 90% and 75% for ERUS. In a large recent European study in 11 centers, MR showed an agreement in T-staging of 57% with 19% overstaging and 24% understaging. It also showed to be very accurate in predicting the extramural depth of tumor ingrowth in the mesorectum, a prognostic factor that is not part of the TNM staging system.[20] MRI is good in identifying large T3 and T4 tumors and invasion of the mesorectal fascia, as described later in this article. Because of the accurate depiction of the tumor mass in large tumors, it is often said that with MRI "what you see is what you get" (**Fig. 2**). Most staging failures with MRI occur in the differentiation between T1 and T2 lesions and between T2 and borderline T3 lesions.[21] A T1 tumor cannot be reliably distinguished from T2 because the submucosal layer is generally not visualized on phased array MRI. Like ERUS, MRI has some difficulty in determining lesions on the border of T2 and T3 with a desmoplastic reaction.[22]

Circumferential Resection Margin

The CRM is the lateral or radial resection margin created by the surgeon. A positive CRM is defined as a closest distance of 1 mm or less between tumor and resection margin, as this represents the optimal prognostic cutoff point. The importance as a prognostic factor and as a parameter of surgical quality has been recognized and confirmed in the past 20 years.[4] The ideal plane of resection in a total mesorectal excision is just outside the mesorectal fascia, and a positive CRM can be the result of inadequate total mesorectal excision (TME) surgery or an advanced tumor that comes close to or invades the mesorectal fascia. The first problem is one of surgical technique, whereas the second is a matter of preoperative identification and adequate neoadjuvant treatment of advanced tumors. For centers that use only a long course of chemoradiation as a neoadjuvant treatment, the distance of the tumor to the

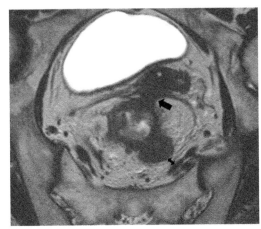

Fig. 2. MRI perpendicular to the long axis of the tumor shows a large tumor, with a posterior component that comes close to but does not invade the mesorectal fascia (*small arrow*), and an anterior component that extends through the mesorectal fascia and invades the uterus (*large arrow*).

mesorectal fascia is usually not very important in the preoperative decision process, as all tumors that extend beyond the muscular wall are considered candidates for a long course of chemoradiation, providing an opportunity for downsizing. For centers that also use a short course of 5 × 5 Gy and immediate surgery, this is different. Although it has been shown that 5 × 5 Gy is a very efficient and cost-effective way to prevent local recurrences in many patients, it is much less effective when the tumor comes close to or invades the mesorectal fascia.[23] These tumors should be identified and treated with a long course of chemoradiation and a long interval to provide down-sizing. Regardless of the neoadjuvant treatment strategies, it is important for the surgeon to know the exact anatomic relation of the tumor to the mesorectal fascia and the surrounding structures to obtain a complete resection, and in advanced cases it can be very valuable to have the images available in the operating room.

With ERUS it is very difficult to identify the mesorectal fascia in patients with a "threatened CRM," except when it shows invasion of vagina, prostate, or seminal vesicles. Many single-center studies have shown that MRI is highly accurate for the prediction of an involved CRM (see **Fig. 2**).[22,24–26] The results of a systematic review confirm the high performance of MRI, showing a sensitivity for the prediction of an involved CRM varying between 60% and 88% and specificity between 73% and 100%.[27] The subsequent large European multicenter Mercury study showed an accuracy of 91% with a negative predictive value of 93% for patients who underwent immediate surgery and 77% accuracy and 98% negative predicitve value after a long course of (chemo)radiation.[28] Two European centers that use a short course of radio-therapy as a treatment option report a decrease in the number of positive margins after the incorporation of MRI in the discussion of all patients with rectal cancer in multidisciplinary meetings.[29,30]

Nodal Stage

Nodal disease is one of the most important risk factors for both local and distant recurrence, and is generally considered an indication for neoadjuvant therapy. Identifying nodal disease with imaging remains, however, difficult because size criteria used on its own result in only a moderate accuracy. Lymph nodes with a diameter of 10 mm or larger are invariable malignant, but most involved nodes are smaller than 5 mm.[31] In addition to size with 5 mm as a cutoff, ERUS also uses roundness, border irregularity, and hypoechoic nature as criteria for malignancy (**Fig. 3**). The pooled sensitivity and specificity of ERUS in a recent meta-analysis based on 35 studies was about 75%, and another meta-analysis of CT, ERUS, and MRI showed that the receiver operating characteristic (ROC) curves were only moderate.[27,32] In the comparative meta-analysis, ERUS performed slightly better than CT or MRI, most likely because of the use of criteria other than size alone. For MRI, the same criteria as on ERUS of roundness and border irregularity, and heterogeneous signal have been found to provide additional accuracy over size alone (**Fig. 4**).[33,34] This can be of help in evaluating nodes that are larger than 5 mm, but a reliable characterization in smaller nodes is not possible. The practical difficulties in nodal staging with the standard imaging methods are illustrated by a recent multicenter report in which T3N0 tumors, staged with ERUS or MRI, were found to be node positive at histology in 22%, despite preoperative chemoradiation.[35]

MR techniques and sequences are continuously improving, and with modern, more powerful, machines, new sequences, and lymph node–specific MR contrast agents the accuracy is likely to improve. An example of a contrast agent is ultrasmall superparamagnetic particles of iron oxide (USPIO), that have been reported to provide a higher accuracy for lymph node characterization in a variety of cancers.[36] This has been confirmed in small pilot rectal cancer node studies, but unfortunately USPIO is not approved by the Food and Drug Administration or European Medicines Agency (EMEA).[37,38] There are many preliminary reports on new MR diffusion sequences in a number of cancer types, but it remains to be awaited if this will improve nodal staging.[39]

How does one work in practice with a suboptimal accuracy of preoperative lymph node imaging? An extreme approach is to disregard the imaging data on nodal status and to give neoadjuvant treatment in most patients, accepting overtreatment rather than undertreatment. This strategy exposes all patients to the side effects of radiotherapy on sexual, urinary, and defecatory function, whereas only a few patients

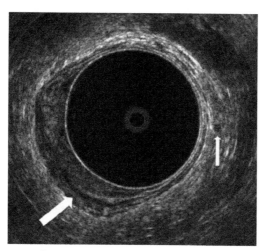

Fig. 3. ERUS of a tumor that grows into the dark hypoechoic layer that represents the muscular wall, without obvious ingrowth in the mesorectal fat, classified as T2. The small node is difficult to classify, but the round aspect and the echogeneity similar to the tumor suggest an involved lymph node. (*Courtesy of* Dr Martin R. Weiser, New York, NY.)

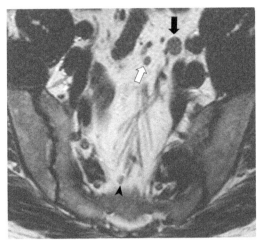

Fig. 4. MRI showing a malignant enlarged round lymph node (*black arrow*), and 2 lymph nodes smaller than 5 mm (*black arrowhead* and *white arrow*) that are difficult to classify with all present imaging techniques.

benefit from improved local control. Another approach is to take into account the prevalence of nodal metastases according to the T stage and to give neoadjuvant therapy for T3 lesions, regardless of nodal imaging results, but not for T2N0 lesions.[35] It can even be argued that the small-volume nodal disease that is easily missed by imaging is prognostically less important for local recurrence and may be controlled by good TME surgery that removes the entire mesorectum, without neoadjuvant therapy.[40] This strategy is further supported by evidence from 2 large European trials of the lack of survival benefit of radiotherapy when good TME surgery is performed.[23,41] Although there are no real data to support or refute any of the previously mentioned approaches, the most practical strategy seems to rely on the information on lymph node staging in the preoperative decision making, keeping in mind the limitations. Nodes that are 5 mm and larger, with a more round than oval shape, that are heterogeneous, and/or have an irregular border should be considered malignant. Whenever these criteria are absent on EUS or MRI for any of the visualized nodes, the nodal status can be considered negative, knowing there is an overall 20% false negative rate. Erring on the safe side, large tumors can be treated with neoadjuvant therapy irrespective of the nodal status. In addition to the standard treatment with TME, there is a small group of patients with a superficial tumor where the surgeon is considering a local excision, a procedure with minimal morbidity and mortality but with a small risk of leaving behind involved lymph nodes in the mesorectum. Accurate selection of node-negative disease would be of help in the selection for this procedure, but unfortunately the smaller the primary tumor the smaller the lymph node metastases, and the lower the accuracy of imaging.[42] It is therefore prudent to select only patients with a low a priori chance for nodal metastases, such as small, well-differentiated T1 lesions, or patients with a high operative risk, and to discuss the oncological risk with the patient.

EXPERTISE, AVAILABILITY, AND COST

It is generally agreed that there is a learning curve for staging with ERUS, and this may explain the lower accuracy in multicenter studies.[11,43,44] There are many technical aspects and details in the performance and interpretation that require attention, and ERUS is therefore considered more operator dependent than MR. In experienced hands, an interobserver variation of 10% to 15% has been reported in T staging.[15] A good overview of the technique and pitfalls is given by Edelman and Weiser.[9] For MRI, it is important to obtain good standard high-resolution sequences, and not to make unnecessary sequences that can be confusing, such as fat suppression. The use of coils has evolved from endorectal coils, with good anatomic delineation of the bowel wall but a small field of view, to whole body coils with less accurate T staging, and then to the present standard of phased array pelvic coils providing high-resolution images. The details of high-resolution MR techniques can be found in radiological literature.[21] Although there is a small learning curve for the interpretation of MR images, the multicenter Mercury study and our own experience showed that the accuracy can be good outside the expert centers.[28]

ERUS has the advantage over MRI that the equipment is less costly and that it can be readily used in the office, immediately providing information that is important for further treatment planning. MRI on the other hand has the advantage over ERUS that the images can be more easily interpreted and read by other radiologists and clinicians. The images can also be used by radiotherapists for planning the radiotherapy fields and by surgeons to guide the resection in advanced cases.

SUMMARY

ERUS and MRI should be seen more as complementary rather than competitive techniques. Each has its own strengths and weaknesses. ERUS is better in showing the tumor extent in small superficial tumors, whereas MRI is superior in imaging the more advanced tumors. The choice of imaging technique depends also on the amount of information that is required for choosing certain treatment strategies, like the distance to the mesorectal fascia for a short course of preoperative radiotherapy. For lymph node imaging, both techniques are at present only moderately accurate, although this could change with advances in new MR techniques.

REFERENCES

1. Cunningham D, Atkin W, Lenz HJ, et al. Colorectal cancer. Lancet 2010; 375(9719):1030–47.
2. Sauer R, Becker H, Hohenberger W, et al. Preoperative versus postoperative chemoradiotherapy for rectal cancer. N Engl J Med 2004;351(17):1731–40.
3. Gunderson LL, Sargent DJ, Tepper JE, et al. Impact of T and N substage on survival and disease relapse in adjuvant rectal cancer: a pooled analysis. Int J Radiat Oncol Biol Phys 2002;54(2):386–96.
4. Nagtegaal ID, Quirke P. What is the role for the circumferential margin in the modern treatment of rectal cancer? J Clin Oncol 2008;26(2):303–12.
5. NIH consensus conference. Adjuvant therapy for patients with colon and rectal cancer. JAMA 1990;264(11):1444–50.
6. Marijnen CA, Nagtegaal ID, Kapiteijn E, et al. Radiotherapy does not compensate for positive resection margins in rectal cancer patients: report of a multicenter randomized trial. Int J Radiat Oncol Biol Phys 2003;55(5):1311–20.
7. Hildebrandt U, Feifel G, Schwarz HP, et al. Endorectal ultrasound: instrumentation and clinical aspects. Int J Colorectal Dis 1986;1(4):203–7.
8. Beynon J, Foy DM, Roe AM, et al. Endoluminal ultrasound in the assessment of local invasion in rectal cancer. Br J Surg 1986;73(6):474–7.

9. Edelman BR, Weiser MR. Endorectal ultrasound: its role in the diagnosis and treatment of rectal cancer. Clin Colon Rectal Surg 2008;21(3):167–77.

10. Schaffzin DM, Wong WD. Endorectal ultrasound in the preoperative evaluation of rectal cancer. Clin Colorectal Cancer 2004;4(2):124–32.

11. Harewood GC. Assessment of publication bias in the reporting of EUS performance in staging rectal cancer. Am J Gastroenterol 2005;100(4):808–16.

12. Bipat S, Glas AS, Slors FJ, et al. Rectal cancer: local staging and assessment of lymph node involvement with endoluminal US, CT, and MR imaging—a meta-analysis. Radiology 2004;232(3):773–83.

13. Marusch F, Koch A, Schmidt U, et al. Routine use of transrectal ultrasound in rectal carcinoma: results of a prospective multicenter study. Endoscopy 2002; 34(5):385–90.

14. Ptok H, Marusch F, Meyer F, et al. Feasibility and accuracy of TRUS in the pre-treatment staging for rectal carcinoma in general practice. Eur J Surg Oncol 2006;32(4):420–5.

15. Garcia-Aguilar J, Pollack J, Lee SH, et al. Accuracy of endorectal ultrasonography in preoperative staging of rectal tumors. Dis Colon Rectum 2002;45(1):10–5.

16. Kauer WK, Prantl L, Dittler HJ, et al. The value of endosonographic rectal carcinoma staging in routine diagnostics: a 10-year analysis. Surg Endosc 2004;18(7): 1075–8.

17. Adams WJ, Wong WD. Endorectal ultrasonic detection of malignancy within rectal villous lesions. Dis Colon Rectum 1995;38(10):1093–6.

18. Kim JC, Yu CS, Jung HY, et al. Source of errors in the evaluation of early rectal cancer by endoluminal ultrasonography. Dis Colon Rectum 2001;44(9): 1302–9.

19. Starck M, Bohe M, Simanaitis M, et al. Rectal endosonography can distinguish benign rectal lesions from invasive early rectal cancers. Colorectal Dis 2003; 5(3):246–50.

20. MERCURY Study Group. Extramural depth of tumor invasion at thin-section MR in patients with rectal cancer: results of the MERCURY study. Radiology 2007; 243(1):132–9.

21. Beets-Tan RG, Beets GL. Rectal cancer: review with emphasis on MR imaging. Radiology 2004;232(2):335–46.

22. Beets-Tan RG, Beets GL, Vliegen RF, et al. Accuracy of magnetic resonance imaging in prediction of tumour-free resection margin in rectal cancer surgery. Lancet 2001;357(9255):497–504.

23. Peeters KC, Marijnen CA, Nagtegaal ID, et al. The TME trial after a median follow-up of 6 years: increased local control but no survival benefit in irradiated patients with resectable rectal carcinoma. Ann Surg 2007;246(5):693–701.

24. Bissett IP, Fernando CC, Hough DM, et al. Identification of the fascia propria by magnetic resonance imaging and its relevance to preoperative assessment of rectal cancer. Dis Colon Rectum 2001;44(2):259–65.

25. Blomqvist L, Machado M, Rubio C, et al. Rectal tumour staging: MR imaging using pelvic phased-array and endorectal coils vs endoscopic ultrasonography. Eur Radiol 2000;10(4):653–60.

26. Peschaud F, Cuenod CA, Benoist S, et al. Accuracy of magnetic resonance imaging in rectal cancer depends on location of the tumor. Dis Colon Rectum 2005;48(8):1603–9.

27. Lahaye MJ, Engelen SM, Nelemans PJ, et al. Imaging for predicting the risk factors—the circumferential resection margin and nodal disease—of local recurrence in rectal cancer: a meta-analysis. Semin Ultrasound CT MR 2005;26(4):259–68.

28. MERCURY Study Group. Diagnostic accuracy of preoperative magnetic resonance imaging in predicting curative resection of rectal cancer: prospective observational study. BMJ 2006;333(7572):779.
29. Beets-Tan RG, Lettinga T, Beets GL. Pre-operative imaging of rectal cancer and its impact on surgical performance and treatment outcome. Eur J Surg Oncol 2005;31(6):681–8.
30. Burton S, Brown G, Daniels IR, et al. MRI directed multidisciplinary team preoperative treatment strategy: the way to eliminate positive circumferential margins? Br J Cancer. 2006;94(3):351–7.
31. Wang C, Zhou Z, Wang Z, et al. Patterns of neoplastic foci and lymph node micrometastasis within the mesorectum. Langenbecks Arch Surg 2005;390(4):312–8.
32. Puli SR, Reddy JB, Bechtold ML, et al. Accuracy of endoscopic ultrasound to diagnose nodal invasion by rectal cancers: a meta-analysis and systematic review. Ann Surg Oncol 2009;16(5):1255–65.
33. Brown G, Richards CJ, Bourne MW, et al. Morphologic predictors of lymph node status in rectal cancer with use of high-spatial-resolution MR imaging with histopathologic comparison. Radiology 2003;227(2):371–7.
34. Kim JH, Beets GL, Kim MJ, et al. High-resolution MR imaging for nodal staging in rectal cancer: are there any criteria in addition to the size? Eur J Radiol 2004; 52(1):78–83.
35. Guillem JG, Diaz-Gonzalez JA, Minsky BD, et al. cT3N0 rectal cancer: potential overtreatment with preoperative chemoradiotherapy is warranted. J Clin Oncol 2008;26(3):368–73.
36. Will O, Purkayastha S, Chan C, et al. Diagnostic precision of nanoparticle-enhanced MRI for lymph-node metastases: a meta-analysis. Lancet Oncol 2006;7(1):52–60.
37. Koh DM, Brown G, Temple L, et al. Rectal cancer: mesorectal lymph nodes at MR imaging with USPIO versus histopathologic findings—initial observations. Radiology 2004;231(1):91–9.
38. Lahaye MJ, Engelen SM, Kessels AG, et al. USPIO-enhanced MR imaging for nodal staging in patients with primary rectal cancer: predictive criteria. Radiology 2008;246(3):804–11.
39. Sugita R, Ito K, Fujita N, et al. Diffusion-weighted MRI in abdominal oncology: clinical applications. World J Gastroenterol. 2010;16(7):832–6.
40. Cecil TD, Sexton R, Moran BJ, et al. Total mesorectal excision results in low local recurrence rates in lymph node-positive rectal cancer. Dis Colon Rectum 2004; 47(7):1145–9 [discussion: 1149–50].
41. Sebag-Montefiore D, Stephens RJ, Steele R, et al. Preoperative radiotherapy versus selective postoperative chemoradiotherapy in patients with rectal cancer (MRC CR07 and NCIC-CTG C016): a multicentre, randomised trial. Lancet 2009; 373(9666):811–20.
42. Landmann RG, Wong WD, Hoepfl J, et al. Limitations of early rectal cancer nodal staging may explain failure after local excision. Dis Colon Rectum 2007;50(10): 1520–5.
43. Orrom WJ, Wong WD, Rothenberger DA, et al. Endorectal ultrasound in the preoperative staging of rectal tumors. A learning experience. Dis Colon Rectum 1990;33(8):654–9.
44. Badger SA, Devlin PB, Neilly PJ, et al. Preoperative staging of rectal carcinoma by endorectal ultrasound: is there a learning curve? Int J Colorectal Dis 2007; 22(10):1261–8.

Optimal Management of Small Rectal Cancers: TAE, TEM, or TME?

Julio Garcia-Aguilar, MD, PhD*, Alicia Holt, MD

KEYWORDS

- Rectal cancer • Local excision • Transanal excision
- Transanal endoscopic microsurgery • Total mesorectal excision
- Neoadjuvant therapy

The ultimate goal of the treatment of rectal cancer is to cure the disease while preserving function and quality of life. Total mesorectal excision (TME), the surgical removal of the rectum and its mesorectal envelope, is the accepted standard approach for the treatment of rectal cancer.[1] Patients with tumors located in the middle or upper rectum often undergo an anterior or low anterior resection, preserving the anal sphincter, whereas patients with distal tumors require a complete abdomino-perineal resection of the rectum, resulting in permanent colostomy. Patients with early-stage (stage I) rectal cancer who undergo this aggressive surgical approach benefit from a high cure rate, with 5-year survival rates reported between 87% to 90%.[2] TME, however, is a major operation that is accompanied by significant mortality (1%–6%) and considerable morbidity. Anastomotic leakage is reported in 5% to 15% of patients undergoing low rectal anastomosis, and genitourinary dysfunction occurs in up to 30% to 40% of patients. Functional disturbances, including bowel urgency, tenesmus, soiling, and fecal incontinence, are also commonly reported, as is depression, developing in 10% to 32% of patients. These sequelae often persist and have a significant impact on quality of life.[3–6] Nonetheless, the associated morbidity and mortality of this surgical intervention are currently justified by the oncologic control provided by this approach.

Local excision (LE) has always been an accepted alternative in patients unfit for radical surgery because of advanced age or comorbid conditions. More recently, LE has been explored as an alternative to TME in selected patients with early-stage rectal cancer. It is appealing because it is less invasive, alleviates the need for a colostomy or the distressing sequelae related to low colorectal anastomosis, and results in low

---

Department of Surgery, City of Hope, 1500 East Duarte Road, Duarte, CA 91010, USA
* Corresponding author.
E-mail address: jgarcia-aguilar@coh.org

Surg Oncol Clin N Am 19 (2010) 743–760
doi:10.1016/j.soc.2010.08.002

morbidity and mortality. But LE alone results in higher rates of local recurrence that, albeit occasionally salvageable by TME, could ultimately compromise long-term survival.[7] Consequently, LE as a curative surgical approach for early rectal cancer has been treated with caution and has yet to gain widespread acceptance. The conventional transanal excision (TAE) is the most widely used approach for LE, but transanal endoscopic microsurgery (TEM) is gaining popularity as a possible alternative, particularly for tumors of the upper rectum that cannot be reached by standard TAE.[8]

The oncologic benefits of neoadjuvant chemoradiation (CRT) observed in patients with locally advanced rectal cancer treated with TME has hastened interest in investigating whether or not CRT could play a role in reducing recurrence after LE in patients with early rectal cancer. Several recent studies suggest that if chemotherapy and radiation therapy are given before LE, the risk of recurrence drops to a level comparable with TME.[9] Although still controversial, LE in combination with preoperative CRT may, therefore, have an expanding role in the treatment of early-stage rectal cancer.

The expansion of colorectal cancer screening programs is increasing the proportion of patients diagnosed with early rectal cancer. The aging of the population is increasing the proportion of high-risk elderly patients with early-stage rectal cancers who may benefit from a less-morbid surgical treatment. These changes probably explain why, in spite of the paucity of information about the advantages of LE compared with TME, the proportion of patients having LE has increased in recent years.[10] The aim of this review is to analyze the current literature to try to identify rectal cancer patients who may benefit from LE.

PATIENT SELECTION CRITERIA FOR LOCAL EXCISION

The ideal candidates for LE, either by TAE or TEM, are patients with rectal cancers localized to the bowel wall, meaning tumors that do not penetrate beyond the muscularis propria and have not metastasized to the perirectal nodes. Because most of the mesorectum is left relatively undisturbed during LE, any tumor cells left in the perirectal fat or the mesorectal lymph nodes may lead to local recurrence and compromised survival. Unfortunately, preoperative clinical findings and imaging studies are not completely accurate in assessing the depth of tumor invasion of the rectal wall and the status of the mesorectal lymph nodes, and patient selection remains one of the most important barriers to the adoption of LE.

Clinical Preoperative Evaluation

Although tumor stage remains the most important criteria for patient selection for LE, several gross features, such as tumor mobility, size, morphology, and distance from the anal verge, should also be taken into consideration.[11,12] Digital rectal examination and proctoscopy provide surgeons with useful information about the tumor and the patient, which is essential for the treatment decision making.[11] Patients with large and fixed tumors can be immediately excluded from consideration for LE. Although tumor size is not a good predictor of depth of invasion or nodal metastasis, patients with tumors larger than 4 cm in diameter or involving more than 40% of the circumference of the rectum are poor candidates for LE.[12–15] The mobility of a tumor on digital rectal examination also provides clues about its depth of invasion.[11] Distinguishing tumor invasion within individual layers of the rectal wall, however, is beyond the capabilities of a clinical examination. Patients with tethered or fixed tumors, which probably invade into the perirectal fat or surrounding tissue, are poor candidates for LE. Tumor morphology and distance from the anal verge do not have independent prognostic value when stratified by tumor stage.[16–19] Distance from the anal verge, however, is important for patient selection. LE is favored in patients with lower lesions because there is a higher risk for permanent colostomy or poor functional results if they are treated with restorative TME.

Radiologic Preoperative Staging

Techniques, such as CT scan and surface coil MRI, are useful for evaluating the abdomen for distant spread and assessing locally advanced tumors. The new-generation CT and MRI are able to detect tumor invasion outside the bowel wall and predict the relationship of the tumor with the circumferential margins[20,21]; however, they do not provide sufficient resolution of the layers of bowel wall to distinguish between a T1 and a T2 lesion or between a polyp and a T1 lesion. Only endorectal ultrasound (ERUS) and endorectal coil MRI can provide this level of detail. Either of these studies should, therefore, be performed in the evaluation of any patients considered for LE.[22,23]

In a systematic review of 53 studies, including 2915 patients, Kwok and colleagues[24] reported the accuracy of ERUS to be 87% for T-stage and 74% for lymph node involvement. For MRI with endorectal coil, the corresponding figures were 84% and 82%. In a large meta-analysis with data from 90 publications, Bipat and colleagues[25] found the sensitivity of ERUS and MRI for tumor invasion outside the rectal wall as high as 90% and 82%, respectively, but sensitivity for lymph node metastasis was significantly lower at 67% and 66%, respectively.

The largest single-institution case review of 545 patients suggested that the accuracy of ERUS in determining depth of invasion is significantly lower than previously published.[26] Garcia-Aguilar and colleagues cited an overall ERUS accuracy rate of only 69% (with 18% overstaged and 13% understaged) when compared with pathologic staging. ERUS accuracy tended to increase with advancing T stage. The ERUS accuracy for T1 tumors was 47%, 68% for T2 tumors, and 70% for T3 tumors. The accuracy of ERUS for detecting the presence or absence of metastatic tumor deposits in mesorectal lymph nodes was only 64% in this study.

This study illustrates the inherent biases that plague studies evaluating ERUS or any type of imaging technique for rectal cancer. Because the gold standard against which the imaging study is compared is the final unirradiated pathologic specimen, only those patients who did not undergo preoperative radiation are included in the study. The majority of patients with obvious advanced disease on the ERUS undergo neoadjuvant therapy and some patients with clearly localized lesions are offered LE. With exclusion of both of these groups, those who are left for evaluation are patients with more equivocal findings on the imaging studies. This selection bias has led to an underestimation of the accuracy of ERUS and MRI.

Although conventional 2-D ERUS is one of the most adequate modalities for preoperative staging of rectal cancer, its ability to correctly evaluate the depth of submucosal invasion remains controversial and its efficacy with respect to treatment selection has not been clarified in detail. 3-D ERUS is based on the construction of a 3-D model from the synthesis of a high number of parallel transaxial 2-D images. Recent information suggests that 3-D reconstruction increases the accuracy of ERUS in assessing the depth of rectal cancer submucosal invasion and aids in selecting patients for LE.[27]

Histology

The most important predictor of lymph node metastasis is depth of tumor invasion (T stage).[28–30] Up to 70% of T3/4 tumors and up to 28% of T2 tumors have lymph node metastasis in the mesorectum. An LE with curative intent is not an option for patients with T2 or T3 tumors because of the high risk of leaving cancer cells in the mesorectal lymph nodes. Even for T1 tumors, the risk of nodal metastasis ranges from 10% to 15%,[28–30] still unacceptably high for LE alone. Attempts to further stratify the risk within this group of tumors have included subdivision of the depth of submucosal invasion and identification of signs of aggressive behavior, such as lymphovascular invasion and poor differentiation. Kudo first introduced the concept of dividing the submucosal layer into three levels (sm1, sm2, and sm3).[31] Sm1 indicates tumor invasion into the upper third of the submucosa, sm2 into the middle third, and sm3 into the lower third. Several studies have demonstrated an association of deeper submucosal invasion with increasing risk of lymph node metastases in 0% to 3% for sm1 lesions to 20% to 23% for sm3 lesions.[15,31–33] Kitajima and colleagues[15] also showed on multivariate analysis that submucosal invasion deeper than 1000 μm was associated with a 5-fold increased risk of lymph node spread (odds ratio 5.4).

Several histologic features have also been associated with a more aggressive subset of T1 tumors with a higher propensity for lymphatic and distant spread.[12,30,34] Blumberg and colleagues[28] reported that poor differentiation and lymphovascular invasion were associated with rates of lymph node metastases of 30% and 33% respectively. Willett and colleagues[30] published an actuarial 5-year survival rate of only 79% in early rectal cancer (T1 or T2) when associated with these adverse histologic features compared with 91% in the presence of favorable histology. Tumor budding (defined as isolated cancer cells or nests of cancer cells in normal tissue at the edge of the main tumor) in T1 rectal cancers has been associated with lymph node metastases in 25% of cases and has been predictive of worse survival after TME independent of disease stage.[35–37]

Although the use of histologic criteria is fraught with pitfalls, including sampling error and interobserver variability, the evidence indicates that high-grade and lymphovascular invasion predict a higher risk of lymph node involvement.[19] Other factors, such as depth of submucosal invasion and tumor budding, are less widely used but also suggest an increased risk. The presence of any of these adverse histologic findings after LE should prompt an unequivocal recommendation for further treatment.

In addition to depth of tumor invasion, histologic type, and lymphatic invasion, gender may be a predictive marker for lymph node metastasis in early rectal cancer. Kobayashi and colleagues[38] showed that approximately 1% of men with well-differentiated T1 adenocarcinoma of the lower rectum had lymph node metastasis. Such patients were deemed suitable candidates for LE. In contrast, the rate of lymph node metastasis in women with histologic types other than well-differentiated adenocarcinoma was 30.4%, even when the tumor did not invade the muscularis propria, suggesting that these patients should not undergo LE but rather TME.

TECHNICAL ASPECTS

TAE of rectal tumors, first described by Parks and colleagues,[39] requires a full bowel preparation and perioperative antibiotics. The procedure is performed under general or regional anesthesia and the patient is placed in either jack-knife prone or lithotomy position, depending on the location of the tumor. Use of a pudenal block assists with relaxation of the sphincter as well as postoperative analgesia.

A Lone Star retractor (Lone Star Medical Products, Inc, Stafford, TX, USA) is used to efface the anus and facilitate exposure of the distal rectum. A Pratt bivalve speculum and Sawyer, Hill-Ferguson, or Ferguson Moon retractors are also used to dilate the anus and visualize the tumor within the rectum. Deeper lesions often require the use of narrow Deaver or even Wylie renal vein retractors. Use of a headlamp is essential to provide sufficient illumination of the field.

Electrocautery is used to define a 1-cm circumferential margin around the tumor. Traction sutures can be placed in the normal tissue around the tumor for better exposure and manipulation. Excision must encompass the full thickness of the rectal wall with the dissection extending into the surrounding mesorectal fat. Additional sutures can be placed in the proximal edge of the normal rectum to aid in closure of the defect. Once the specimen is fully excised, it should be oriented and pinned before sending it to pathology. The rectal wall defect is closed transversely and a proctoscopic examination is performed at the end of the procedure to assure the rectum is unblocked. TAE is a safe procedure with minimal morbidity. Postoperative pain and discomfort are usually minor. Patients may eat on the evening of the operation, and most are discharged with 48 hours of the operation. Serious complications, including local sepsis, fecal incontinence, rectovaginal fistula, and rectal stricture, are rare.[9]

TEM has been used successfully in the management of rectal adenoma and in selected cases of rectal carcinoma.[8] It offers a minimally invasive alternative to TAE, with endoscopic magnification and illumination that provide excellent visualization and multiple instruments that allow precise resection and secure suture closure. A 40-mm operating rectoscope is placed and CO_2 is insufflated into the rectum to provide exposure. Special instruments are used through the rectoscope to excise the tumor and close the defect in the rectal wall. The removal of the tumor follows the same guidelines as standard TAE. This technique allows excellent visualization and access for more proximal tumors. Distal lesions are more difficult to excise with TEM because the seal between the rectoscope and the anal canal is insecure and this prevents proper insufflation of the rectum. Like the standard transanal approach, TEM is also a safe procedure with a low rate of complications. Although there has been concern about anal sphincter injury from prolonged stretch, several studies have documented no lasting adverse effect on anorectal function.[8]

Given the inaccuracy of the clinical staging of rectal cancer, underestimation of the level of tumor invasion of the rectal wall is common. Consequently, a partial-thickness excision of the bowel wall (either by TAE or TEM) carries a high risk of positive resection margins in understaged tumors. In a recent study of 424 patients with rectal tumors treated by TEM, Bach and colleagues[40] found that a partial-thickness excision of the bowel wall was associated with a 6-fold increase in the risk of an R1 resection compared with full-thickness excision. A partial excision should only be performed for benign lesions provided the surgeon is prepared to perform a full-thickness excision or a TME for unsuspected invasion in the surgical specimen. All other patients should have a full-thickness excision. LE should always be viewed as an excisional biopsy of the tumor, after which the need for any additional therapy can be determined.[30,31]

RESULTS OF TAE

There are many publications reporting the results of TAE alone for the treatment of rectal cancer, but most of them are small, single-institution case series. The reported local recurrence rates range from 0 to 28% for T1 lesions and 11% to 45% for T2 lesions, whereas 5-year survival rates range from 74% to 90% for T1 lesions and 55% to 75% for T2 lesions. The wide variation in reported outcomes probably reflects differences in patient selection, intent of surgery, and surgical technique (reviewed by Kim and colleagues[7]).

Several retrospective case series and reviews of population-based registries have compared the outcomes of patients with early rectal cancer treated by TAE and

TME (**Table 1**).[10,41–46] Although these studies have intrinsic selection bias with patients who had TAE being older and having tumors closer to the anal verge compared with TME patients who tended to be younger and had larger tumors, they provide useful information regarding the outcomes of patients with early rectal cancer. All of them report higher local recurrence rates and lower overall survival for tumors treated by TAE compared with TME. These differences are larger in patents with T2 tumors, but in most series the differences in outcomes between TAE and TME also reach statistical significance for T1 tumors. In one of the largest series published so far, You and colleagues[10] evaluated a cohort of 35,179 patients from the National Cancer Database treated for stage I rectal cancer between 1989 and 2003 and compared the results of 765 patients treated by LE (601 with T1 tumors and 164 with T2 tumors) with 1359 selected patients treated by standard surgical resection. After adjusting for tumor and patient characteristics, the 5-year local recurrence rate after LE was found to be significantly higher than after TME for both T1 tumors (12.5% vs 6.9%; $P = .003$) and T2 tumors (22.1% vs 15.1%; $P = .01$). The 5-year overall survival was not influenced by the type of procedure performed for T1 tumors (77.4% for LE vs 81.7% for TME; $P = .09$) but was lower after LE compared with TME for T2 tumors (67.6% vs 76.5%; $P = .01$). In this series, no operative mortality was reported for either type of surgery, but patients treated by TME had a 14.6% complication rate compared with 5.6% for patients treated by TAE. In the data from the Swedish Rectal Cancer Registry, the complication rate for LE was 11.5% for patients treated with LE compared with 35.4% for patients treated by low anterior resection and 20.6% for patients treated by abdominoperineal resection.[42]

The results of these studies suggest that bearing in mind the selection bias inherent to retrospective case series, TAE is an inferior oncologic operation compared with TME because it results in higher local recurrence rates. There is also a clear trend toward better survival after TME, in particular for patients with T2 tumors. Although patients treated by TAE tend to be older, the rate of complications is lower compared with younger patients treated by TME. Other important outcomes for the treatment of these patients, such as bowel and urinary function, proportion of patients left with a stoma, and quality of life, were not captured in these studies.

RESULTS OF TEM

Most reports on the outcomes of TEM for rectal cancer have the same problems described for TAE: small retrospective case series with variable selection criteria, differences in technique, the use of neoadjuvant therapy, definitions of outcomes, and length of follow-up. The reported rates of local recurrence range from 0 to 10% for T1 tumors and 7% to 29% for T2 tumors, survival from 79% to 100% for T1 tumors, and 70% to 95% for T2 tumors. These results are not significantly different compared with patients treated with TAE.[8]

Bach and colleagues[40] recently reported the outcomes of 424 patients with rectal cancer treated with TEM and entered into a national database. A positive resection margin occurred in 11%, 22%, and 42% of T1, T2, and T3 tumors, respectively. A total of 146 (35%) patients received additional therapy, either CRT or TME, and the remaining 278 (65%) patients were observed. The investigators performed a multivariate analysis to identify predictors of recurrence. Three histologic variables, depth of tumor invasion, maximum tumor diameter, and the presence of lymphovascular invasion predicted local recurrence-free survival. Patients who were observed after TEM (with or without postoperative radiation) were fifteen times more likely to develop

Table 1
Results of retrospective series comparing TAE with TME for T1 rectal cancer

Series	T Stage	TAE					TME					
		N	Mort	Comp	LR	OS	N	Mort	Comp	LR	OS	FU
Hazard et al[41] (2009)	1	418 (855[a])	NR	NR	NR	71%	1035 (3465[b])	NR	NR	NR	84%*	3.9
	2	155				58%	2005				77%*	
You et al[10] (2007)	1	601	0.5%	5.6%	8.2%	77%	22	1.8%	14.6%	4.3%*	82%	>5
	2	164			12.6%	68%	83			7.2%*	77%*	
Folkesson et al[42] (2007)	1,2	256 (643[a])	NR	11.5%	7.2%	95%	1802 (7891[b])	NR	35%–41%	2.8%	84%–94%	2.5
Bentrem et al[43] (2005)	1	151	NR	NR	15%	89%	168	NR	NR	3%	93%	4.3
Endreseth et al[44] (2005)	1	35	2.9%	NR	12%	70%	256	2.3%	NR	6%*	80%*	2.8
Nascimbeni et al[45] (2004)	1	70	NR	NR	6.6%	72%	74	NR	NR	2.8%	90%*	8.1
Mellgren et al[46] (2000)	1	69	NR	NR	18	72%	30	NR	NR	0	80%	4.8
	2	39			47	65%	123			6	81%	

Abbreviations: Comp, complications; FU, follow-up; LR, local recurrence; Mort, mortality; NR, not reported; OS, overall survival.
* Signifies statistical significance.
[a] Total number of patients treated by TAE.
[b] Total number of patients treated by TME.

a local recurrence than those who were converted to TME based on unfavorable histologic criteria. Of the 63 patients who had a TME, only five patients developed tumor recurrence, one local and four distant. Their prediction model indicated that patients with pT1 tumors less than 3 cm in diameter that were well or moderately differentiated and had no lymphovascular invasion had a 93% probability to be free of disease at 3 years. For T1 tumors of other hystopathological criteria and T2 tumors, the 3-year local recurrence-free survival was much lower. They concluded that TEM should be considered an "excisional diagnostic biopsy" and that only patients with T1 tumors, with negative margins and a favorable histology should be considered for observation. Patients with T2 tumors or adverse histopathology should be converted to TME.

Two prospective randomized trials and four case series have compared the results of TEM with TME (**Table 2**) in patients with early rectal cancer.[47–52] In a study published in 1996, Winde and colleagues[47] randomized 50 patients with T1 rectal cancer to either TEM or anterior resection. At a mean follow-up of 46 months, there was no significant difference in the local recurrence rate (4.2% vs 0) or the survival rate (96% vs 96%) between the two groups. Lezoche and colleagues[48] randomized patients with T2N0 rectal cancer to TEM or laparoscopic TME after neoadjuvant CRT. Local recurrence and survival were not different after 84 months of follow-up. The four retrospective case series reported higher local recurrence rates after TEM compared with TME but no significant difference in survival. Mortality and morbidity were lower in patients treated with TEM.

Although the number of patients in the series comparing TEM and TME is smaller than in the studies comparing TAE with TME, the results are similar in the sense that both show a higher recurrence rate, a trend toward decreased survival, and lower morbidity with the LE techniques compared with TME.[47–52]

A purported advantage of TEM over conventional TAE is improved visualization of the tumor, simultaneous instrumentation, and access to tumor located in the mid- or upper rectum which theoretically could translate into more secure resection margins and better oncologic outcomes. There are no prospective studies comparing both techniques, however. A recent study from the University of Minnesota compared their experience with TAE and TEM as the only form of therapy for patients with T1 and T2 rectal cancer.[53] It found that resection margins were more often positive in the TAE group (16%) compared with the TEM group (2%). Similar complications were also found in both groups. The rate of local recurrence was higher for patients treated with TAE compared with patients treated with TEM, but the difference did not reach statistical significance. Tumor T stage, resection margin status, use of adjuvant chemotherapy, and tumor distance from the anal verge were the only predictors of local recurrence and disease-free survival in multivariate analysis. Surgical technique, TAE or TEM, was not an independent predictor of outcomes. The investigators conclude that although TEM may be a superior technique for LE in terms of achieving negative resection margins, it does not provide a significant survival advantage compared with TAE.[53]

SALVAGE THERAPY AFTER LOCAL EXCISION

The fundamental risk of choosing LE over TME is the possibility of allowing a curable disease to progress to an incurable state through inadequate treatment. If recurrent or residual disease could be readily detectable and salvage surgery could render a cure, this risk would be minimized. Unfortunately, experiences from several centers indicate that even with careful follow-up, significant tumor progression occurs before residual disease is detected in the form of local recurrence. A large number of patients who

Table 2
Comparison of TEM versus TME for T1 and/or T2 rectal cancer

Series	T Stage	TEM					TME					FU (mon)
		N	Mort	Comp	LR	OS	N	Mort	Comp	LR	OS	
de Graaf et al[49] (2009)	1	80	0%	5%	24%*	75%	75	4%	64%	0%	77%	64
Lezoche et al[48] (2007)	2	35	0%	14%	5.7%	94%	35	0%	17%	2.8%	94%	84
Lee et al[50] (2003)	1	52	0%	4.1%	4.1%	100%	22	0%	48%	0%	93%	31–35
	2	22			19.5%*	95%	83			9.4%*	96%	
Langer et al[51] (2003)	1	20 (79[a])	0%	7.6%	10%	NS	18 (27[b])	3.7%	56%	0%	NS	43–21
Heintz et al[52] (1998)	1 (lr)	46	0%	2%	4.4%	79%	34%	6%	15%	2.9%	81%	42–52
	1 (hr)	12	0%	10%	33%	62%	11%	0%	30%	18.2%	69%	
Winde et al[47] (1996)	1	24	0%	29%	4.1%	96%	26	0%	58%	0%	96%	46

Abbreviations: Comp, complications; FU, follow-up; lr/hr, lowrisk/high-risk tumors based on presence of poor differentiation or lymphovascular invasion; LR, local recurrence; Mon, months; Mort, mortality; NS, not stated; OS, overall survival.
* P<.05.
[a] Total number of patients treated by TEM.
[b] Total number of patients treated by TME.

recur with unresectable tumors and those who are able to undergo curative resections often require extended resections. Five-year survival rates are below 50%, which is in marked contrast to the 85% to 90% survival rates seen in stage I rectal cancer patients treated initially with TME.[54–57]

In the University of Minnesota series reported by Friel and colleagues,[54] patients were methodically followed after LE with proctoscopy and ERUS every 4 months. Despite this intensive surveillance, 93% of patients who recurred presented with more advanced disease (stage II or higher). Curative resection (R0) was possible in only 79% of the patients, and the disease-free survival rate was only 59% at 39 months of follow-up. In the Memorial Sloan-Kettering Cancer Center experience, 94% of patients underwent curative resections, but more than half of the patients required extended pelvic dissections with en bloc resection of surrounding structures.[55] Despite this aggressive approach, the disease-free survival was still only 53% at a median follow-up of 33 months. In the series of Bentrem and colleagues,[43] complete resection was possible in 77% of local recurrences after TAE compared with 50% of local recurrences after TME, but the actuarial 5-year disease free survival was only 58%.

Baron and colleagues[56] compared the results of salvage TME done immediately after local treatment for worrisome tumor characteristics with salvage surgery done after clinically detected local recurrence. Five-year disease-free survival rate was significantly better for those undergoing immediate salvage (94.7% vs 55.5%). A major flaw of this study was that the two groups were not directly comparable. The delayed salvage group consisted of patients who all clearly had recurrent disease whereas the immediate resection group included some patients who would not have recurred even without the TME. Despite this limitation, the results are consistent with the other studies and underscore the lost opportunity for cure when inadequately treated early-stage rectal cancer is allowed to progress. Immediate salvage with TME is recommended for patients who are found to have lesions that signal a high risk of local recurrence ($\geq$T2, adverse histologic features). Hahnloser and colleagues[57] showed that this approach does not result in worse oncologic outcomes when compared with initial TME.

There is a reasonable concern that when an LE has to be converted to TME due to unfavorable histology or positive resection margins, the fascial plane of the mesorectum may be already violated resulting in an R1 TME resection. Although recurrences after TME reoperations after LE have been reported, they are infrequent and immediate salvage TME after TAE or TEM is probably safe.[40]

When deciding between LE and TME, patients need to realize that the tradeoff of lower morbidity for higher mortality risk is real, particularly for T2 tumors. Local recurrence may carry a significant price in terms of extensive salvage operations and decreased survival. These results emphasize the need for careful patient selection if LE is considered a treatment option. In addition, close follow-up is mandatory after LE. Even though Friel and colleagues[54] showed that significant disease progression can occur despite intense surveillance, 81% of the patients in the University of Minnesota cohort were asymptomatic at the time of their diagnosis.[58] Additional delay in diagnosis until the appearance of symptoms would make salvage less feasible.

ADJUVANT CRT AFTER LOCAL EXCISION

Patients found to have unfavorable histopathologic features after LE and who either refuse or are unfit for immediate salvage surgery have been commonly treated with CRT with the intention to reduce the risk of local recurrence. Many individual case series hare reported their results with the use of radiation or CRT after LE for early rectal cancer, but the best available evidence consists of two small prospective trials and a well-designed retrospective cohort study.[59–61]

In an attempt to improve sphincter conservation rates among patients with early low rectal cancer, the Radiation Therapy Oncology Group conducted a multi-institutional, phase II, prospective trial evaluating adjuvant CRT therapy after LE.[59] Based on the final histopathologic findings, patients were divided into three groups. The first group had T1 lesions with favorable histologic features and secure margins. This group received no further treatment and was only observed. The second group had T1 tumors with unfavorable histology or lesions greater than or equal to T2. This group received the standard dose of CRT. The third group was same as the second except the resection margins were not secure and this risk factor prompted a higher dose of CRT. After a median follow-up of 6.1 years, local-regional recurrences developed in 16% of the patients (8/65). The risk of recurrence correlated with T stage (T1, 4%; T2, 8%; and T3, 23%) and degree of involvement of the resection margin. For the two groups treated with CRT, the 5-year actuarial freedom from pelvic relapse was 86%. Although the small number of patients does not allow for any firm conclusions, these recurrence rates, especially for T2 and T3 tumors, compare favorably with historical controls treated with TME and suggest a beneficial effect of CRT.

The Cancer and Leukemia Group B conducted a similar prospective multi-institutional trial comparing the outcomes of 59 patients with T1 lesions treated with LE alone and 51 patients with T2 lesions treated with LE and postoperative CRT.[60] At a median follow-up of 7.1 years, the local recurrence rates were 8% for the T1 and 18% for the T2 group. The 10-year actuarial overall and disease-free survival rates were 84% and 75% for T1 and 66% and 64% for T2 group, respectively. These results were considered comparable with the survival data reported for stage I disease by the National Cancer Database.[60]

Chakravarti and colleagues[61] retrospectively compared patients with T1/T2 rectal cancer treated by LE alone with those treated by LE plus adjuvant radiation therapy (LE + XRT). As expected, a significantly higher percentage of T2 tumors and T1 tumors with unfavorable histologic features were found in the radiation therapy group. Overall, there was no difference in the 5-year local recurrence and disease-free survival rates between the two groups. In a subgroup analysis of only the high-risk patients (T1 with lymphovascular invasion/high-grade or T2 tumors), however, the local control rate was substantially better with the addition of postoperative radiation therapy (LE, 37%, vs LE + XRT, 85%). There was also an improvement in disease-free survival although this difference did not reach statistical significance (37% vs 58%; $P = .29$).

In summary, despite the lack of randomized controlled trials to show the benefit of adjuvant CRT or radiation therapy after LE, there seems to be a trend toward lower recurrence rates and higher disease-free survival with adjuvant therapy when compared with LE alone. Adjuvant therapy after LE may be more beneficial in T2 or T3 tumors, or higher-grade tumors.

LOCAL EXCISION AFTER NEOADJUVANT CRT

In recent years, several retrospective studies have examined the effect of preoperative CRT in patients with early rectal cancer who were candidates for LE, reporting on tumor response rate, recurrence, and survival (**Table 3**).[62–69] Mohiuddin and colleagues[62] were the first to report their experience with 30 T3 rectal cancer patients treated with preoperative radiotherapy followed by LE. A total of 11 (36%) patients had

Table 3
CRT before local excision

	Tumor Stage			Recurrence	
	T2	T3	pCR	Local ± Distant	Survival
Garcia-Aguilar et al[72] (2010)	77	—	43%	NR	NR
Yeo et al[69] (2010)	—	11	73%	18%	89%
Callender et al[68] (2010)	—	47	49%	21%	79%
Lezoche et al[67] (2008)	35	—	32%	9%	94%
Bonnen et al[66] (2004)	—	26	54%	11%	86%
Schell et al[64] (2002)	—	11	73%	9%	100%
Ruo et al[63] (2002)	6	4	30%	20%	78%
Kim et al[65] (2001)	26		73%	4%	92%
Mohiuddin et al[62] (1994)	18	40	30%	10%	83%

Abbreviation: NR, not reported.

a pathologic complete response (pCR) and a 5-year recurrence rate of 10% and survival rate of 83% were reported. Since then, other retrospective case series have reported variable results in patients with T2 and T3 rectal cancer. Although these studies are limited by small numbers and mixed populations of patients, they suggest that preoperative CRT can be successfully used to downstage tumors before LE and that T2 and even T3 tumors treated with CRT and LE have lower local recurrence rates compared with LE alone.

Bonnen and colleagues[66] compared the outcomes of 26 patients who underwent LE after CRT with 405 patients who underwent TME after the same preoperative CRT regimen during the same period of time. They reported a pCR rate of 54% (11 out of 26 patients) after preoperative CRT and LE on T3-staged tumors and 35% of patients with microscopic residual disease. The 5-year local recurrence rate in the LE patients was 6% and overall survival was 86% compared with 8% and 81% for the TME group. Patients in the LE group, however, had less advanced disease and better response to CRT: all but one patient in the LE group had uT3N0 preoperative stage whereas 57% of TME patients were staged as uT3N1. Callander and colleagues[68] have recently updated the results of this series after a median follow-up of 63 months. Ten-year actuarial local recurrence was not significantly different between the LE and TME groups (10.6% vs 7.6%, respectively; $P = .52$), and no significant difference in survival was found between the groups. In spite of the selection bias favoring LE, these results suggest that CRT before LE may be an appropriate treatment for selected patients with T3 rectal cancers.

These results contrast with other series that have reported the results of unselected patients with clinically and ultrasound-staged T3N0 rectal cancer treated by neoadjuvant CRT and TME. Guillem and colleagues[70] found that 41 (22%) of 188 of their ERUS/MRI-staged T3N0 rectal cancer patients had metastatic lymph nodes in the mesorectum after preoperative CRT. Lombardi and colleagues[71] have also reported a 28% positive node rate among 32 patients with clinically staged T3N0 rectal cancer patients treated with neoadjuvant therapy and surgery. This discrepancy between the node positivity in T3N0 rectal cancer treated by CRT and TME (22% to 28%) and the low recurrence rate reported by Bonnen and colleagues (6%) could be explained by differences in accuracy of the preoperative staging between series. The possibility that some of the cancer cells present in the lymph nodes at the time of surgery could have regressed with a longer follow-up, however, cannot be excluded. Alternatively, it is possible that some patients in Bonnen and colleagues' series may still have clinical occult cancer cells in the mesorectal nodes at the time of analysis that may lead to clinical recurrences with longer follow-up.

Lezoche and colleagues[48] conducted a prospective randomized trial comparing TEM and TME after neoadjuvant CRT in patients with T2N0 rectal cancer. The overall pCR rate was approximately the same in both groups (35%). In the most recent update of this trial with a median follow-up of 84 months, only two of 35 (5.7%) patients had local recurrence in the TEM group and only 1 of 35 (2.8%) in the TME group (2.8%). Disease-free survival after 84 months of median follow-up was similar (94%) in both groups. Although this study was clearly underpowered, it provides the strongest evidence supporting a role for CRT and TEM for patients with T2N0 rectal cancer.

To further explore the role of neoadjuvant CRT and LE for rectal cancer, the American College of Surgeons Oncology Group (ACOSOG) conducted the Z6041 study, a multicenter, phase II, clinical trial using neoadjuvant CRT followed by LE in patients with ultrasound-staged T2N0 rectal cancer aimed at determining disease-free survival at 3-years, pCR rate, CRT-related toxicity, and perioperative surgical complications (**Fig. 1**). The study closed to accrual on November of 2009 after accruing 90 patients. Preliminary results presented as an abstract reported a 98% resection rate with negative margins.[72] Among 77 eligible patients who underwent LE, 49 (64%) tumors were downstaged (ypT0-1), and 4 patients (5%) had ypT3 tumors. Five LE specimens contained lymph nodes; one T3 tumor had a positive node. The pCR rate was 43%, in line with what has been published in other series of early rectal cancers treated with CRT and LE.[72] Although these preliminary data are encouraging, the efficacy of CRT and LE will be realized when the long-term oncologic and quality-of-life data can be examined.

The preliminary results of the ACOSOG Z6041 study highlight the limitations of patient selection for the implementation of the CRT plus LE approach for early rectal cancer. Patients for this study were eligible if they had a T2N0 by ERUS. Although some of the pathologic T1 tumors may have been downstaged by the CRT, it is possible that some may have been overstaged by ERUS. What is known is that 4 of 77 patients were understaged with respect to bowel wall invasion. Consequently, similar to patients treated with TAE or TME alone, LE after CRT should be considered a full-thickness excisional biopsy and the final decision regarding the need for additional treatment should be based on the evaluation of the surgical specimen.

Similar to what occurs with unirradiated specimens, there is a correlation between the level of tumor infiltration in the rectal wall and the risk of nodal metastasis in rectal

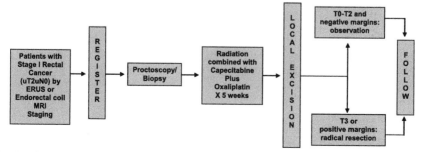

Fig. 1. ACOSOG Z6041 study schema.

cancer patients after CRT. The deeper the residual tumor in the bowel wall, the higher the risk of positive nodes in the mesorectum. For patients with ypT0 tumors—no viable cancer cells in the rectal wall—the reported rate of positive nodes in the mesorectum rages from 0 to 12%. Therefore, LE may not guarantee cure even in patients with ypT0 tumors after CRT. What needs to be defined is the risk of nodal metastasis in patients with clinically N0 tumors who become ypT0 after CRT.

SUMMARY

TME remains the gold standard for rectal cancer because it provides superior onco-logic outcomes compared with LE. LE can be offered as an alternative for carefully selected patients; however, it must be emphasized that even in ideal patients LE does not achieve equivalent results regarding oncologic outcomes compared with TME. With LE, patients trade a higher cancer cure rate for a lower risk of mortality and lower morbidity.

Patients with early rectal cancer confined to the bowel wall without evidence of nodal disease by optimal imaging can undergo LE or TME. If the former is chosen, a full-thickness excision of the section of the rectal wall containing the tumor should be performed. This can be performed by TAE or TEM depending on tumor location and surgeon expertise. Final pathologic features of the tumor and the resection margins should determine the need for further treatment. Only T1 tumors with favor-able histologic features and negative resection margins can be observed. Patients with other tumors—T1 lesions with adverse features and T2 and more advanced tumors—who are aiming for a curative treatment should be offered salvage TME. A patient's age, comorbid condition, as well as wishes and expectations should also be taken into consideration in the decision-making process.

The role of CRT and LE in the treatment of rectal cancer is still under study. Prelim-inary data accumulated thus far suggest that many early rectal cancers respond to CRT, that the probability of negative resection margins is higher than with TAE or TEM alone, and that CRT and LE may provide similar oncologic results compared with TME. Similar to LE alone, final treatment decisions should be based on the pathology examination of the surgical specimen. Tumor response to CRT provides additional information about the biologic behavior of the tumor, but as with LE alone, accurate preoperative staging for adequate patient selection is essential.

ACKNOWLEDGMENTS

The authors thank Nicola Solomon, PhD, for assistance in writing and editing the manuscript.

REFERENCES

1. Heald RJ, Moran BJ, Ryal RDH, et al. Rectal cancer. The Basingstoke experience of total mesorectal excision, 1978–1997. Arch Surg 1998;133:894–9.
2. Blumberg D, Paty PB, Picon AI, et al. Stage I rectal cancer: identification of high-risk patients. J Am Coll Surg 1998;186(5):574–9 [discussion: 579–80].
3. Peeters KC, van de Velde CJ, Leer JW, et al. Late side effects of short-course preoperative radiotherapy combined with total mesorectal excision for rectal cancer: increased bowel dysfunction in irradiated patients—a Dutch colorectal cancer group study. J Clin Oncol 2005;23(25):6199–206.

4. Lange MM, den Dulk M, Bossema ER, et al. Cooperative Clinical Investigators of the Dutch Total Mesorectal Excision Trial. Risk factors for faecal incontinence after rectal cancer treatment. Br J Surg 2007;94(10):1278–84.
5. Lange MM, Maas CP, Marijnen CA, et al. Cooperative Clinical Investigators of the Dutch Total Mesorectal Excision Trial. Urinary dysfunction after rectal cancer treatment is mainly caused by surgery. Br J Surg 2008;95(8):1020–8.
6. Nesbakken A, Nygaard K, Bull-Njaa T, et al. Bladder and sexual dysfunction after mesorectal excision for rectal cancer. Br J Surg 2000;87(2):206–10.
7. Kim E, Hwang JM, Garcia-Aguilar J. Local excision for rectal carcinoma. Clin Colorectal Cancer 2008;7(6):376–85.
8. Suppiah A, Maslekar S, Alabi A, et al. Transanal endoscopic microsurgery in early rectal cancer: time for a trial? Colorectal Dis 2008;10:314–29.
9. Borschitz T, Wachtlin D, Mohler M, et al. Neoadjuvant chemoradiation and local excision for T2-3 rectal cancer. Ann Surg Oncol 2008;15(3):712–20.
10. You YN, Baxter NN, Stewart A, et al. Is the increasing rate of local excision for stage I rectal cancer in the United States justified? A nationwide cohort study from the National Cancer Database. Ann Surg 2007;245(5):726–33.
11. Nicholls RJ, Mason AY, Morson BC, et al. The clinical staging of rectal cancer. Br J Surg 1982;69(7):404–9.
12. Zenni GC, Abraham K, Harford FJ, et al. Characteristics of rectal carcinomas that predict the presence of lymph node metastases: implications for patient selection for local therapy. J Surg Oncol 1998;67(2):99–103.
13. Ueno H, Price AB, Wilkinson KH, et al. A new prognostic staging system for rectal cancer. Ann Surg 2004;240(5):832–9.
14. Kikuchi R, Takano M, Takagi K, et al. Management of early invasive colorectal cancer. Risk of recurrence and clinical guidelines. Dis Colon Rectum 1995; 38(12):1286–95.
15. Kitajima K, Fujimori T, Fujii S, et al. Correlations between lymph node metastasis and depth of submucosal invasion in submucosal invasive colorectal carcinoma: a Japanese collaborative study. J Gastroenterol 2004;39(6):534–43.
16. Papillon J. Intracavitary irradiation of early rectal cancer for cure. A series of 186 cases. Cancer 1975;36(2):696–701.
17. Leong AF, Seow-Choen F, Tang CL. Diminutive cancers of the colon and rectum: comparison between flat and polypoid cancers. Int J Colorectal Dis 1998;13:151–3.
18. Chambers WM, Khan U, Gagliano A, et al. Tumour morphology as a predictor of outcome after local excision of rectal cancer. Br J Surg 2004;91(4):457–9.
19. Nascimbeni R, Burgart LJ, Nivatvongs S, et al. Risk of lymph node metastasis in T1 carcinoma of the colon and rectum. Dis Colon Rectum 2002;45(2):200–6.
20. Muthusamy VR, Chang KJ. Optimal methods for staging rectal cancer. Clin Cancer Res 2007;13(22 Pt 2):6877s–84s.
21. Beets-Tan RG, Beets GL, Vliegen RF, et al. Accuracy of magnetic resonance imaging in prediction of tumour-free resection margin in rectal cancer surgery. Lancet 2001;357(9255):497–504.
22. Puli SR, Bechtold ML, Reddy JB, et al. How good is endoscopic ultrasound in differentiating various T stages of rectal cancer? Meta-analysis and systematic review. Ann Surg Oncol 2009;16(2):254–65.
23. Puli SR, Reddy JB, Bechtold ML, et al. Accuracy of endoscopic ultrasound to diagnose nodal invasion by rectal cancers: a meta-analysis and systematic review. Ann Surg Oncol 2009;16(5):1255–65.
24. Kwok H, Bissett IP, Hill GL. Preoperative staging of rectal cancer. Int J Colorectal Dis 2000;15(1):9–20.

25. Bipat S, Glas AS, Slors FJ, et al. Rectal cancer: local staging and assessment of lymph node involvement with endoluminal US, CT, and MR imaging—a meta-analysis. Radiology 2004;232(3):773–83.
26. Garcia-Aguilar J, Pollack J, Lee SH, et al. Accuracy of endorectal ultrasonography in preoperative staging of rectal tumors. Dis Colon Rectum 2002;45(1): 10–5.
27. Santoro GA, D'Elia A, Battistella G, et al. The use of a dedicated rectosigmoidoscope for ultrasound staging of tumours of the upper and middle third of the rectum. Colorectal Dis 2007;9(1):61–6.
28. Blumberg D, Paty PB, Guillem JG, et al. All patients with small intramural rectal cancers are at risk for lymph node metastasis. Dis Colon Rectum 1999;42(7): 881–5.
29. Sitzler PJ, Seow-Choen F, Ho YH, et al. Lymph node involvement and tumor depth in rectal cancers: an analysis of 805 patients. Dis Colon Rectum 1997I;40(12): 1472–6.
30. Willett CG, Compton CC, Shellito PC, et al. Selection factors for local excision or abdominoperineal resection of early stage rectal cancer. Cancer 1994;73(11): 2716–20.
31. Kudo S. Endoscopic mucosal resection of flat and depressed types of early colorectal cancer. Endoscopy 1993;25(7):455–61.
32. Tytherleigh MG, McC Mortinson NJ. Options for sphincter preservation in surgery for low rectal cancer. Br J Surg 2003;90(8):922–33.
33. Ishizaki Y, Takeda Y, Miyahara T, et al. Evaluation of local excision for sessile-type lower rectal tumors. Hepatogastroenterology 1999;46(28):2329–32.
34. Okabe S, Shia J, Nash G, et al. Lymph node metastasis in T1 adenocarcinoma of the colon and rectum. J Gastrointest Surg 2004;8(8):1032–9 [discussion: 1039–40].
35. Hase K, Shatney C, Johnson D, et al. Prognostic value of tumor "budding" in patients with colorectal cancer. Dis Colon Rectum 1993;36(7):627–35.
36. Wang HS, Liang WY, Lin TC, et al. Curative resection of T1 colorectal carcinoma: risk of lymph node metastasis and long-term prognosis. Dis Colon Rectum 2005; 48(6):1182–92.
37. Hase K, Shatney CH, Mochizuki H, et al. Long-term results of curative resection of "minimally invasive" colorectal cancer. Dis Colon Rectum 1995;38(1):19–26.
38. Kobayashi H, Mochizuki H, Kato T, et al. Is total mesorectal excision always necessary for T1-T2 lower rectal cancer? Ann Surg Oncol 2010;17(4):973–80.
39. Parks AG, Smith R, Morgan CN. Benign tumours of the rectum. In: Smith R, Rob C, Morgan CN, editors. Clinical surgery. London: Butterworths; 1966. p. 541.
40. Bach SP, Hill J, Monson JR, et al. A predictive model for local recurrence after transanal endoscopic microsurgery for rectal cancer. Br J Surg 2009;96(3): 280–90.
41. Hazard LJ, Shrieve DC, Sklow B, et al. Local excision vs. radical resection in T1-2 rectal carcinoma: results of a Study From the Surveillance, Epidemiology, and End Results (SEER) Registry Data. Gastrointest Cancer Res 2009;3(3): 105–14.
42. Folkesson J, Johansson R, Påhlman L, et al. Population-based study of local surgery for rectal cancer. Br J Surg 2007;94(11):1421–6.
43. Bentrem DJ, Okabe S, Wong WD, et al. T1 adenocarcinoma of the rectum: transanal excision or radical surgery? Ann Surg 2005;242(4):472–7 [discussion: 477–9].
44. Endreseth BH, Myrvold HE, Romundstad P, et al. Transanal excision vs. major surgery for T1 rectal cancer. Dis Colon Rectum 2005;48(7):1380–8.

45. Nascimbeni R, Nivatvongs S, Larson DR, et al. Long-term survival after local excision for T1 carcinoma of the rectum. Dis Colon Rectum 2004;47(11):1773–9.
46. Mellgren A, Sirivongs P, Rothenberger DA, et al. Is local excision adequate therapy for early rectal cancer? Dis Colon Rectum 2000;43(8):1064–71 [discussion: 1071–4].
47. Winde G, Nottberg H, Keller R, et al. Surgical cure for early rectal carcinomas (T1). Transanal endoscopic microsurgery vs. anterior resection. Dis Colon Rectum 1996;39(9):969–76.
48. Lezoche G, Baldarelli M, Guerrieri M, et al. A prospective randomized study with a 5-year minimum follow-up evaluation of transanal endoscopic microsurgery versus laparoscopic total mesorectal excision after neoadjuvant therapy. Surg Endosc 2008;22(2):352–8.
49. de Graaf EJ, Doornebosch PG, Tetteroo GW, et al. Transanal endoscopic microsurgery is feasible for adenomas throughout the entire rectum: a prospective study. Dis Colon Rectum 2009;52(6):1107–13.
50. Lee W, Lee D, Choi S, et al. Transanal endoscopic microsurgery and radical surgery for T1 and T2 rectal cancer. Surg Endosc 2003;17(8):1283–7.
51. Langer C, Liersch T, Süss M, et al. Surgical cure for early rectal carcinoma and large adenoma: transanal endoscopic microsurgery (using ultrasound or electrosurgery) compared to conventional local and radical resection. Int J Colorectal Dis 2003;18(3):222–9.
52. Heintz A, Mörschel M, Junginger T. Comparison of results after transanal endoscopic microsurgery and radical resection for T1 carcinoma of the rectum. Surg Endosc 1998;12(9):1145–8.
53. Christoforidis D, Cho HM, Dixon MR, et al. Transanal endoscopic microsurgery versus conventional transanal excision for patients with early rectal cancer. Ann Surg 2009;249(5):776–82.
54. Friel CM, Cromwell JW, Marra C, et al. Salvage radical surgery after failed local excision for early rectal cancer. Dis Colon Rectum 2002;45(7):875–9.
55. Weiser MR, Landmann RG, Wong WD, et al. Surgical salvage of recurrent rectal cancer after transanal excision. Dis Colon Rectum 2005;48(6):1169–75.
56. Baron PL, Enker WE, Zakowski MF, et al. Immediate vs. salvage resection after local treatment for early rectal cancer. Dis Colon Rectum 1995;38(2):177–81.
57. Hahnloser D, Wolff BG, Larson DW, et al. Immediate radical resection after local excision of rectal cancer: an oncologic compromise? Dis Colon Rectum 2005;48(3):429–37.
58. de Anda EH, Lee SH, Finne CO, et al. Endorectal ultrasound in the follow-up of rectal cancer patients treated by local excision or radical surgery. Dis Colon Rectum 2004;47(6):818–24.
59. Russell AH, Harris J, Rosenberg PJ, et al. Anal sphincter conservation for patients with adenocarcinoma of the distal rectum: long-term results of radiation therapy oncology group protocol 89-02. Int J Radiat Oncol Biol Phys 2000;46(2):313–22.
60. Greenberg JA, Shibata D, Herndon JE 2nd, et al. Local excision of distal rectal cancer: an update of cancer and leukemia group B 8984. Dis Colon Rectum 2008;51(8):1185–91 [discussion: 1191–4].
61. Chakravarti A, Compton CC, Shellito PC, et al. Long-term follow-up of patients with rectal cancer managed by local excision with and without adjuvant irradiation. Ann Surg. 2000;231(4):614.
62. Mohiuddin M, Marks G, Bannon J. High-dose preoperative radiation and full thickness local excision: a new option for selected T3 distal rectal cancers. Int J Radiat Oncol Biol Phys 1994;30(4):845–9.

63. Ruo L, Guillem JG, Minsky BD, et al. Preoperative radiation with or without chemotherapy and full-thickness transanal excision for selected T2 and T3 distal rectal cancers. Int J Colorectal Dis 2002;17(1):54–8.

64. Schell SR, Zlotecki RA, Mendenhall WM, et al. Transanal excision of locally advanced rectal cancers downstaged using neoadjuvant chemoradiotherapy. J Am Coll Surg 2002;194(5):584–90 [discussion: 590–1].

65. Kim CJ, Yeatman TJ, Coppola D, et al. Local excision of T2 and T3 rectal cancers after downstaging chemoradiation. Ann Surg 2001;234(3):352–8 [discussion: 358–9].

66. Bonnen M, Crane C, Vauthey JN, et al. Long-term results using local excision after preoperative chemoradiation among selected T3 rectal cancer patients. Int J Radiat Oncol Biol Phys 2004;60(4):1098–105.

67. Lezoche E, Guerrieri M, Paganini AM, et al. Long-term results in patients with T2-3 N0 distal rectal cancer undergoing radiotherapy before transanal endoscopic microsurgery. Br J Surg 2005;92(12):1546–52.

68. Callender GG, Das P, Rodriguez-Bigas MA, et al. Local excision after preoperative chemoradiation results in an equivalent outcome to total mesorectal excision in selected patients with T3 rectal cancer. Ann Surg Oncol 2010;17(2):441–7.

69. Yeo SG, Kim DY, Kim TH, et al. Local excision following pre-operative chemoradiotherapy-induced downstaging for selected cT3 distal rectal cancer. Jpn J Clin Oncol 2010;40(8):754–60.

70. Guillem JG, Díaz-González JA, Minsky BD, et al. cT3N0 rectal cancer: potential overtreatment with preoperative chemoradiotherapy is warranted. J Clin Oncol 2008;26(3):368–73.

71. Lombardi R, Cuicchi D, Pinto C, et al. Clinically-staged T3N0 rectal cancer: is preoperative chemoradiotherapy the optimal treatment? Ann Surg Oncol 2010;17(3):838–45.

72. Garcia-Aguilar J, Qian S, Thomas CR Jr, et al. Pathologic complete response (pCR) to neoadjuvant chemoradiation (CRT) of uT2uN0 rectal cancer (RC) treated by local excision (LE): results of the ACOSOG Z6041 trial [abstract 3510]. J Clin Oncol 2010;28(Suppl):15s.

Low Anterior Resection: Alternative Anastomotic Techniques

David J. Schoetz Jr, MD[a,b,c,*], Rocco Ricciardi, MD, MPH[a,b]

KEYWORDS

- Rectal cancer • Anterior resection • Proctectomy
- Pouch • Coloplasty • Baker

WORKUP AND EVALUATION

A thorough and comprehensive evaluation of the patient with rectal cancer is critical in order to select optimal surgical therapy. The evaluation includes an assessment of patient suitability for surgery as well as clinical tumor staging. Proctectomy is a difficult procedure for even the fittest of patients, so every effort should be made to optimize patient comorbidities before surgery. Thus, a complete clinical assessment is essential to gauge comorbidities and define operative risk as well as to explore the patient's goals in treatment. An assessment of sphincter function and preexisting issues related to fecal incontinence or prior sphincter injury is also essential in assessing suitability for sphincter preservation.

The patient with rectal cancer should undergo a thorough evaluation of the colon and rectum with colonoscopy to assess the primary tumor and to identify and remove synchronous polyps or to localize and biopsy synchronous cancers.[1] When possible, the distal border of the tumor is tattooed if chemoradiation is to be provided preoperatively, because determining the distal extent of the tumor is often difficult following neoadjuvant therapy. Given the high rates of complete pathologic response, it is not uncommon for a patient to have no visible lesion at the time of proctectomy, rendering the preoperative tattoo critical. Colonoscopy is important for identification of synchronous cancers or other large unresectable polyps, which may alter treatment plans. If colonoscopy is incomplete, imaging with a double-contrast barium enema or virtual

Funding support: Not applicable.
Disclosure: Not applicable.
[a] Department of Colon and Rectal Surgery, Lahey Clinic, 41 Mall Road, Burlington, MA 01805, USA
[b] Tufts University School of Medicine, MA, USA
[c] Department of Medical Education, Graduate Medical Education, MA, USA
* Corresponding author. Department of Colon and Rectal Surgery, Lahey Clinic, 41 Mall Road, Burlington, MA 01805.
E-mail address: David.J.Schoetz@Lahey.org

Surg Oncol Clin N Am 19 (2010) 761–775
doi:10.1016/j.soc.2010.07.002
1055-3207/10/$ – see front matter © 2010 Elsevier Inc. All rights reserved.

colonoscopy is a suitable alternative.[1] If preoperative surveillance of the proximal colon is not possible, intraoperative colonoscopy can be considered.

Accurate local and regional staging with radiographic imaging is also essential to select the most appropriate treatment regimen for patients with rectal cancer. Local staging begins with rectal examination and proctoscopy or flexible sigmoidoscopy to determine the location of the tumor in relationship to the anal sphincter mechanism. Imaging is a critical component of the workup for rectal cancer, not only to assess T and N stage but also to provide information regarding contiguous spread from the primary rectal cancer to adjacent nearby structures such as the sphincter mechanism, lateral pelvic sidewalls, prostate, seminal vesicles, vagina, bladder, and sacrum. The precise extent of such local invasion can be assessed by several modalities such as magnetic resonance imaging (MRI), endorectal ultrasonography, or pelvic computed tomography (CT) scanning. MRI is one of the more accurate methods to assess depth of rectal cancer invasion, thereby accurately predicting potentially involved circumferential margins as well as enlarged lymph nodes.[2] Although endorectal ultrasonography characterizes depth of penetration (T stage) and is useful in assessing involvement of the anterior structures such as the vagina or prostate/seminal vesicles, this technique is not as effective in assessing lateral extrarectal spread.[3] MRI is also well suited for identifying poor prognostic features such as extramural spread greater than 5 mm, extramural venous invasion, nodal involvement, and peritoneal infiltration.[4] Given the importance of accurate local staging, MRI has increasingly become the preferred diagnostic imaging study for rectal cancer.[5]

In addition to local staging, evaluation for distant disease is similarly critical, because detection of metastases may completely change the approach to a rectal cancer. The lungs and liver are the most common organs to harbor distant metastases. Patients with rectal cancer should undergo evaluation with either chest radiography or CT to exclude pulmonary metastases. Abdominal CT or right upper quadrant MRI is also recommended for evaluation of liver metastases. Although metastases can occur to other organs, additional imaging is recommended only if symptoms or findings on physical examination raise suspicion of other sites of spread. At this time the role of other imaging modalities, such as positron emission tomography scanning, in the primary evaluation of colorectal cancers is not yet completely understood.

TEAM APPROACH (NEOADJUVANT THERAPY)

There are several treatment strategies available to the patient with rectal cancer, which depend on the preoperative evaluation outlined earlier. Regardless of stage, most proximal rectal cancers are intraperitoneal and biologically mimic the clinical behavior of colon cancers. Conversely, the treatment of mid to distal, locally advanced rectal cancers is variable, generally relying on multimodal protocols that are formulated based on tumor stage and other factors delineated during the preoperative assessment. The aim of this article is to specifically focus on locally advanced disease, so the authors do not include here a discussion of surgical approaches to superficial tumors of the rectum amenable to local excision or proximal cancers of the rectum. Local excision is a viable option for early-stage tumors of the rectum, and these approaches are outlined in more detail in other articles.

Surgical approaches to locally invasive distal rectal cancer are complex because these tumors have a high risk for positive circumferential (radial) or distal margins leading to a high risk for locoregional recurrence. Thus, neoadjuvant chemoradiotherapy is often recommended to patients with locally advanced mid to distal rectal cancer, because it is associated with decreased local recurrence when compared with postoperative therapy.[6] In a large prospective, multicenter, randomized study, local recurrence was significantly lower and tumor downstaging improved in the preoperative chemoradiotherapy group as compared with the postoperative adjuvant therapy group.[6] Despite equivalent 5-year disease-free survival and overall survival rates, the decreased local recurrence rate in this trial has led the National Comprehensive Cancer Network[7] to recommend consideration for preoperative chemoradiation (long course) for all patients with T3 or T4 rectal cancers. Advantages of neoadjuvant chemoradiotherapy include a high rate of complete pathologic response, lower proportion of positive circumferential margins, and a higher likelihood of sphincter-sparing surgery.

SURGICAL TECHNIQUE

Patients with locally invasive nonmetastatic rectal cancer are generally best treated by a radical resection, a form of either low anterior resection (LAR) or abdominoperineal resection (APR). Anterior resection may be further subdivided into high, low, and ultralow techniques. A high anterior resection generally involves partial proctectomy with intraperitoneal anastomosis, whereas a low resection includes complete mobilization of the rectum and an extraperitoneal anastomosis. Ultralow resection refers to transaction of the rectum just above the pelvic floor with an anastomosis at or just above the top of the puborectalis muscle. Regardless of whether the resection is high or low, the tumor itself with satisfactory proximal, distal, and radial margins must be excised. The decision regarding reestablishment of gastrointestinal tract continuity is then dictated by the conditions after tumor removal as well as other key details obtained during workup.

Initial Steps and Preparation

The patient and bowel is prepared as per the surgeon's preferences. Despite the data demonstrating similar patient outcomes with or without mechanical bowel preparation, our practice is to provide a bowel preparation for all patients with potential for low anastomosis and diverting stoma. Diverting a low anastomosis with a column of feces in the remnant colon seems illogical and thus it is preferred to mechanically cleanse all of these patients. In addition, all patients with distal rectal tumors should have consideration for preoperative stoma marking by a qualified enterostomal therapist. Patient education as well as an understanding of optimal stoma placement is a critical component of the preoperative evaluation as well as the postoperative course. Ureteral stents are also considered for large, bulky, upper tumors or inflammatory lesions.

In the operating room, the patient is placed in the lithotomy position and a bladder catheter is introduced. Before incision, a digital rectal examination and rigid proctoscopy are performed to empty the rectum and reassess the location of the rectal cancer. During examination under anesthesia, anal sphincter involvement is assessed as well as the response of the tumor to chemoradiation. As previously described in the preoperative evaluation section, to facilitate tumor localization the distal border of the tumor is tattooed before initiating chemoradiation to facilitate tumor identification in the operating suite. In addition, prior to incision the distal rectum is washed with either hypotonic solution or a Betadine solution to reduce the potential for tumor shedding.

It is critical that appropriate instruments and other equipment are available for the optimal conduct of the operation. First, headlights and/or lighted retractors are prepared for visualization deep in the pelvis. Self-retaining retractors are often necessary, as are long and deep retractors such as the St Mark retractor and the Wylie renal vein retractors. In addition to long retractors, the surgeon should have access to long instruments and cautery extenders. Most importantly, the operating surgeon will find that the assistance of a second surgeon is critical during the deep pelvic dissection.

Mobilization

After entry into the abdomen, a thorough exploration is performed to exclude metastases or other potential anatomic variations. The small bowel is then packed into the upper abdomen and the patient is placed in Trendelenburg position. The dissection begins along the line of Toldt as the peritoneum is incised along the left side of the sigmoid and descending colon as far caudad as the splenic flexure. The left ureter and gonadal vessels are identified early and preserved. The colon mobilization extends proximally to the transverse colon as adhesions to the spleen are divided and the splenic flexure is mobilized inferiorly.

Pedicle Ligation

The inferior mesenteric artery is best exposed by retracting the rectosigmoid anteriorly and to the left. The vascular pedicle can then be taken either proximally, that is, high ligation of the inferior mesenteric artery as it branches from the aorta, or more distally, that is, low ligation of the artery just distal to the left colic artery. At present, there is not enough evidence to encourage use of one technique over the other. However, it has been found that for an anastomosis to the mid or distal rectum, division and ligation of inferior mesenteric vein is often critical to assure adequate mobility of the descending colon. Following ligation of the vascular pedicle, it is most convenient to divide the colon with a linear stapler.

Total Mesorectal Excision

The standard approach for low rectal cancers involves total mesorectal excision (TME). This technique involves dissection along the areolar plane between the visceral fascia of the mesorectum and the parietal fascia of the pelvic walls. Proper TME removes the intact mesorectum with all of the lymph nodes and the rectum en bloc. For more proximal rectal cancers, a partial mesorectal excision can be performed with a distal margin of 3 to 5 cm. To perform the procedure, the rectosigmoid is retracted anteriorly and inferiorly toward the pubis to expose the avascular plane posterior to the rectum. Sharp incision of this avascular plane with proper rectosigmoid traction permits air to enter the areolar tissues posteriorly and lateral to the rectum. During the retrorectal portion of the mesorectal dissection, the hypogastric nerves are identified at the sacral promontory with an aim toward autonomic nerve preservation. The presacral (Waldeyer) fascia is then divided under direct vision as the dissection proceeds distally to the level of the coccyx. The rectum is mobilized in a posterior-to-lateral direction, with care taken to maintain the integrity of the endopelvic fascial envelope encasing the bilobed mesorectum.

To expose the anterior dissection plane, the angle of the Trendelenburg position is reduced or the patient can even be placed in reverse Trendelenburg. The dissection proceeds in an anterolateral plane by opening the cul-de-sac. Deep pelvic retractors are used to protect the seminal vesicles and prostate in men or the vagina in women. The surgeon then encounters Denonvilliers' fascia in the midline anteriorly. In Heald's[8,9] classic description of TME, Denonvilliers' fascia is considered the most anterior limit of the mesorectum and is thus removed with the specimen. Denonvilliers' fascia is similarly excised for circumferential and anterior rectal tumors to ensure a negative circumferential margin. For posterior tumors, the visceral fascia propria of the rectum is followed and the parietal Denonvilliers' fascia is spared to minimize risk of injury to the nearby periprostatic pelvic nerves.

The importance of the circumferential resection margin (CRM) on oncologic outcome has gained considerable attention. An involved CRM is associated with increased likelihood of local recurrence and shortened survival.[10–12] In fact, studies reveal that local recurrence occurred in 22% of patients with a positive CRM but only 5% if the CRM was negative for cancer.[10,13] Much of the focus on circumferential margins has come from a better understanding of surgical technique and in particular the TME technique, which has led to improvements in oncologic outcomes.[14] Workshops have been held in various European nations for surgeons to acquire the skills needed to perform TME and for pathologists to learn how to properly assess the rectal cancer specimen, including the mesorectum, as described by Quirke and colleagues.[10]

Distal Margin

The choice between sphincter-sparing and APR must be based on assessment of the adequacy of the distal and circumferential margins after complete rectal mobilization. In the past, a distal margin of 5 cm was considered an oncologic necessity, leading to sphincter sacrifice in most cases of distal rectal cancer. However, an evolved understanding of the biology of tumor spread has allowed modification of traditional surgical techniques. It is now known that distal intramural spread of tumor is rare, as is distal lymphatic spread[15] below the gross extent of the tumor. With this knowledge, attempts to decrease the acceptable distal margin and preserve gastrointestinal continuity without sacrificing cancer cure have gained traction.

Because all radical resections for rectal cancer should rely on the same proximal, lateral, and radial mobilization, the decision to perform an anastomosis is based on the ability to obtain clear margins as well as a tension-free, well-vascularized anastomosis. Patient preferences to avoid a permanent colostomy, and adequate preoperative comprehension of altered postoperative bowel function must be taken into account, but ultimately oncologic principles should not be compromised. Occasionally, circumstances arise in which the cancer is larger than anticipated or is extending into tissues outside the boundary of the usual TME dissection. In such cases, a more extensive operation than was originally planned is appropriate to provide curative intent. In these circumstances, performance of an anastomosis may seem technically difficult. Similarly, when the dissection must continue into the anal mucosa or internal sphincter, the ability to reconstruct with an anastomosis may also seem challenging. In these situations, intersphincteric dissection and ultralow anastomosis has been described as a sphincter-preserving alternative to APR for cancers within 5 cm of the anal verge. For those tumors with partial invasion into the upper anal canal, at least a portion of the internal sphincter muscle must be removed to improve the radial and/or distal resection margin. Schiessel and colleagues[16] recently updated a growing experience combining TME and autonomic nerve preservation with a total or partial intersphincteric resection at the intersphincteric groove. When the tumor invades into the external sphincter or levator ani muscle, sphincter preservation with anastomosis is generally contraindicated, although some investigators have described partial external sphincter excision as well. At this time, long-term functional and oncologic results are lacking for this type of radical resection.

Other options for sphincter preservation include coloanal anastomosis as described by Parks and Percy.[17] In this operative technique a pull-through type of anastomosis is performed between the sigmoid or descending colon and the distal rectum or anal canal through the anus. Despite a paucity of data, Parks and Percy advocated for mucosectomy with direct anastomosis that unfortunately leads to mucosectomized anal wall that is nonvisible for surveillance endoscopically. In the original description, 76 patients underwent this operation with recurrence and survival rates comparable to historical controls of patients with similar tumors treated by more traditional operations. All patients had a temporary loop colostomy to protect the anastomosis and none of the patients received radiation therapy. Unfortunately, functional abnormalities were common, as patients described both excess stool frequency and irregularity. There has not been a randomized prospective study regarding the desirability of routine mucosectomy with coloanal pull-through procedures.

The aim in reconstructing a patient following anterior resection is to obtain a 1-cm distal margin and a clean circumferential margin by staying within the mesorectal fascia. Functional outcomes are probably better with preservation of the internal sphincter and avoidance of mucosectomy, but adequate tumor clearance (both intramural and mesorectal) is absolutely critical before an anastomosis can be considered. If clearance is adequate and anal sphincter function appropriate, the surgeon may consider anastomosis. At the time of surgery, options for handling the distal rectum or upper anus include right-angle clamps or staplers. If an open purse-string suture is to be placed in the distal rectal cuff, a right-angle clamp is placed distally on the anorectum and the specimen is divided between 2 clamps. Alternatively, if a double-stapled reconstruction is planned instead, a transverse anastomosis stapler is placed distally. The stapler is fired and the rectum divided, leaving a closed rectal cuff for subsequent anastomosis. The surgeon should then examine the resected specimen to assess the radial and distal margins and evaluate the integrity of the mesorectal and rectal dissection. If the margins are inadequate, the mesorectum has been violated, or perforation of the rectum has occurred, local recurrence is a major concern. The treatment plan may have to be altered to reduce the risk of recurrence.

Anastomosis

Following tumor extirpation, consideration is given to creating an anastomosis that is nonporous while closely approximating the function of the normal rectum. Traditionally, the straight end-to-end anastomosis has been the default anastomotic method following radical proctectomy, but postoperative function is considered poor especially in the setting of a very low anastomosis. Thus, several other techniques have been developed including the side-to-end (Baker technique), colon J-pouch, and coloplasty. Although indications for use of one anastomosis over another are lacking, each anastomotic technique has supporters while particular patient characteristics might sway the surgeon to choose one particular type. In addition, all of the anastomotic techniques can be hand sewn or stapled, depending on the surgeon's preference as well as the oncologic need for mucosectomy.

End-to-end

The straight end-to-end colorectal anastomosis is the traditional choice after radical proctectomy for cancers of the rectum. The technique can be stapled or hand sewn but with improvements in overall technique and staplers in particular, the anastomosis became easier to perform with any of the circular staplers now available. The advantages of the end-to-end anastomosis are ease of construction and ability to mate the 2 ends with minimal tension or excessive mobilization. However, an increased capacity to easily establish the anastomosis lower and lower in the pelvis has led to 2 problems: increased incidence of anastomotic leaks and anterior resection syndrome, that is, bowel dysfunction that is characterized by excessive passing of stool, clustering of bowel movements, and incontinence. These issues have led many surgeons to consider alternative methods for low pelvic anastomosis such as the side-to-end anastomosis, coloplasty, and colon J-pouch procedures.

Side-to-end

One of the earliest reports of the side-to-end (Baker) anastomosis was published in 1950 by Baker.[18] This anastomotic method was originally described as a "low end to side rectosigmoid anastomosis"; however, with the advent of staplers, surgeons began to use the technique at lower and lower levels in the pelvis. In addition, as the functional consequences of end-to-end anastomosis became evident, the Baker anastomosis became an alternative to the more technically complex colon J-pouch or coloplasty procedure.

The side-to-end procedure is performed with either hand-sewn techniques or the circular stapler. In the very low anastomosis, however, the authors prefer to staple this reconstruction. The anastomosis is performed by placing the anvil of the stapler into the divided distal end of the descending colon. Then, the trocar of the anvil is gently brought out of the antimesenteric side of the colon at a length of 4 to 5 cm from the cut end of the distal colon (proximal bowel). Although some surgeons find it important to place a purse-string suture at the point in which the trocar pierces the bowel wall, this is not necessary. The open end of the descending colon is then closed with either a linear stapler or suture sealed. Lastly, the circular stapler is brought out of the top of the acute Hartmann to anastomose the side of the colon to the end of the anus or rectum.

Colon J-pouch

The colon J-pouch was described separately by Lazorthes and colleagues[19] and Parc and colleagues[20] as a reconstruction modification that reduces the severity of the anterior resection syndrome. Thus, the pouch was developed to improve the bowel function results of patients with low pelvic anastomoses. Although functional improvements were initially believed to be caused by increased storage capacity for stool, it has become more accepted that the functional advantage of the colon J-pouch is not a result of its reservoir capacity but a change in colonic motility.[21] As with the other techniques, this reconstruction method can similarly be performed with hand-sewn or stapled techniques.

The colon J-pouch construction requires several technical components to achieve a functional pouch. In addition to an adequate sphincter mechanism and healthy proximal bowel, the intestine must be mobile enough and the pelvis must be wide enough so that the pouch reaches the lower pelvis. Thus, most often the descending colon must be completely mobilized as well as freeing the distal transverse colon and splenic flexure from its attachments. Often, the left colic artery and inferior mesenteric vein must be ligated to provide adequate length. After adequate mobilization, the descending colon is folded into a J configuration with the efferent limb of the J-pouch no larger than 5 to 6 cm, as efferent limb lengths are associated with difficulty in evacuation.[22] The pouch is constructed by inserting a linear cutting stapler through an apical colotomy and approximating the antimesenteric surfaces. The linear staple line is then inspected for bleeding and a decision is made as to the method of construction, either hand sewn or stapled. If a circular stapler technique is chosen, the anvil of the circular stapler is placed into the prior colotomy and secured in place with a purse-string suture. The circular stapler is then inserted gently through the acute Hartmann and an end-to-pouch anastomosis constructed between the J-pouch and anus. If the decision is to hand sew, then the colotomy at the apex of the J-pouch is left open and brought down to the top of the anus. A hand-sewn one-layer anastomosis can then be performed from below with proper retraction via the transanal route.

Coloplasty

The coloplasty technique was developed in response to difficulties related to the suitability of some patients for colon J-pouches. The coloplasty pouch is a simple technique that permits a tension-free anastomosis without significant alteration of colon anatomy. This technique is particularly advantageous in patients with a thick mesocolon and/or a narrow pelvis who are poor candidates for J-pouch reconstruction. This commonly encountered scenario was identified in 25% of patients in a study in which pelvic anatomy or colon thickness rendered them unsuitable candidates for colonic J-pouch.[23]

The coloplasty procedure is similar to a pyloroplasty, in which a colotomy is performed with an 8- to 10-cm long antimesenteric incision at a point 5 to 6 cm from the divided end of the descending colon. If the decision is to staple the anastomosis, the anvil of the circular stapler is placed into the colotomy and brought out from the divided end of the colon before closure of the coloplasty. The colotomy is closed in a transverse direction, perpendicular to the antimesenteric border, with either absorbable sutures or a linear stapler. An end-to-end anastomosis is then performed with the circular stapler.

Which Anastomosis and When?

The anterior resection syndrome is commonly experienced following LAR and, as discussed earlier, is characterized by frequent bowel movements, fecal urgency, stool fragmentation, incontinence, or a combination of all of these symptoms. Poor gastrointestinal function was the impetus for the development of new pelvic reconstruction techniques that increase neorectal capacity and improve function.[22–24] However, the functional advantages of these new reconstruction methods, particularly the colon J-pouch, were most discernible early on after operation.[25,26] More recently, a randomized controlled trial comparing functional outcomes of coloplasty, colon J-pouch, or a straight anastomosis revealed significant and lasting benefits for the colon J-pouch as compared with the straight anastomosis or coloplasty reconstruction.[27]

The end-to-end anastomosis is preferred for reconstruction proximal to 7 to 8 cm, as no studies have established a benefit to the colon J-pouch at levels proximal to 8 cm[24] However, The colon J-pouch is preferred for low anastomoses and generally a small pouch, that is, 5 or 6 cm in length rather than 10 cm, is constructed.[22] For particularly low anastomoses, the colon J-pouch reconstruction is the anastomosis of choice, as data reveal that the greatest functional improvements are observed in patients with a colon J-pouch anastomosis 4 cm or less from the anal verge.[27–29] In addition to the previously described randomized, controlled trial that demonstrated the long-term functional superiority of colon J-pouch,[27] the long-term functional benefits of colon J-pouch were reinforced in a meta-analysis evaluating bowel function outcomes.[29]

The authors like the side-to-end anastomosis for low pelvic anastomosis whereby the colon J-pouch is technically difficult or in which the side-to-end anastomosis is anatomically easier to construct. Small studies have demonstrated equivalency of the side-to-end anastomosis and the colon J-pouch[29] 2 years after LAR. These data reveal no significant difference in surgical outcome between colon J-pouch and side-to-end anastomosis when the outcomes of blood loss, hospital length of stay postoperative complications, reoperations, or functional results are analyzed.[28] However, this study did favor the colon J-pouch in one category: at 6 months, the ability to evacuate the bowel in less than 15 minutes was worse among patients with side-to-end anastomosis.[28] Unfortunately, comparative data are lacking and given the technical ease of side-to-end anastomosis, this procedure has become an excellent alternative to pouch reconstruction.

The coloplasty was also developed to overcome the difficulty of the pouch reconstruction in a patient with a narrow pelvis and thick mesentery. However, the functional results have been mixed, and other data reveal an increased incidence of anastomotic leak after coloplasty reconstruction as compared with colon J-pouch reconstruction.[26] In the meta-analysis detailed earlier, the authors concluded that further study is necessary to determine the role of coloplasty in coloanal anastomotic strategies.[29] It is the authors' practice to use the coloplasty for those situations in which a side-to-end anastomosis or colon J-pouch is not feasible. This technique may be of some value in those patients who require some form of reconstruction but need the length provided with an end-to-end anastomosis to reach the top of the distal bowel. Further data are needed before this reconstruction procedure can be recommended as preferable to the simple end-to-end anastomosis.

Anastomotic Method

Hand-sewn anastomosis

Any of the earlier reconstruction procedures can be hand sewn in 1 or 2 layers with either interrupted or continuous sutures. A hand-sewn colorectal anastomosis is generally constructed from the abdominal incision. Sutures are placed evenly at approximately 4 to 5 mm from the previous suture and without excessive tension to avoid tissue ischemia. For more difficult lower pelvic anastomoses, it is easiest to place the sutures on the distal side first and then parachute the proximal bowel down to the distal end. The mucosa can be inverted by using Lembert sutures or by laying the knots inside the lumen.

For anastomoses at the top of the anus, with or without mucosectomy, a hand-sewn coloanal anastomosis may be performed transanally. This procedure is generally performed in lithotomy with the aid of an abdominal operator. A retractor such as the Parks instrument is necessary for proper visualization. Then the colon is passed through the anal cuff and full-thickness bites of an absorbable suture are placed every 5 mm. The authors elect to divert these patients with a proximal loop ileostomy for at least 2 months.

Double purse-string stapled anastomosis

The double purse-string stapled anastomosis technique is performed with the distal bowel open. Surgeons sometimes force the stapler to the top of the rectum thereby producing rectal lacerations or, alternatively, perform an anastomosis to the anterior midrectum because the stapler is not easily passable to the top of the acute Hartmann. Thus, the advantages for this technique include the capability of the surgeon to manipulate the circular stapler in a cephalad direction to the top of a particularly curvy rectum. First, a continuous monofilament suture is purse-stringed along the open rectal or anal cuff and a second purse-string suture is placed in the colon. The circular stapler is placed through the anus and can be advanced to the top of the rectum by introducing a digit through the open rectal cuff and gently guiding the stapler to the top of the cuff. The anastomotic pouch or neorectum can then be stapled as per routine and the anastomosis air tested for leaks as described now for the double-stapled technique.

Double-stapled anastomosis

The double-stapled technique has the advantage of reducing potential fecal contamination by stapling the rectal cuff. First, a transverse stapler is placed below the cancer to divide the rectum from the specimen. Then a monofilament purse-string suture is placed around the cut edge of the distal lower colon. A circular stapler anvil is then inserted into the descending colon while the purse string is tied. The authors elect to air-leak test the stapled acute Hartmann or distal rectal stump to reduce the possibility of unidentified air leak from the transverse staple line corners. If an air leak is identified from the acute Hartmann, then the circular stapler obturator is brought out through the rent in the staple line. If there is no air leak, the circular stapler is advanced through the rectum to the top of the rectal cuff and the obturator is opened in the center of the transverse staple line. The mobilized descending colon and anvil is then mated to the top of the circular stapler, closed, and fired, resulting in the finished anastomosis. The anastomosis is then air tested with a proctoscope while the anastomosis is under irrigant.

Role of Temporary Fecal Diversion

The incidence of anastomotic complications following low pelvic anastomosis is highest as the anastomosis draws closer to the anus. In fact, the risk of anastomotic complications is reported to range from 4.9% to 17% in the literature.[30] In addition, a history of radiation therapy, immunosuppression, and diabetes increases the risk of anastomotic complications. Given that the sequelae of a leaking anastomosis remain a major source of morbidity and mortality after reconstruction for proctectomy, some surgeons have taken to routinely diverting patients following a low anastomosis. Others have recommended temporary fecal diversion in the setting of low anastomosis and after preoperative irradiation, to reduce the consequences of a leak.[31] Initially, proximal fecal diversion was believed to diminish the morbidity resulting from leakage and reduce the likelihood of an emergency reoperation.[31] However, recently there have been 2 meta-analyses that have demonstrated a reduced clinical anastomotic leak rate in patients with defunctioning stoma[32,33] as compared with no fecal diversion. Fecal diversion is considered for patients with a low colorectal anastomosis if (1) they have undergone preoperative radiation therapy, (2) have a pelvic pouch or coloplasty reconstruction, or (3) technical issues are experienced during reconstruction.

APR

The APR procedure involves en bloc resection of the rectosigmoid, the rectum, and the anus along with the surrounding mesentery, mesorectum, and perianal soft tissues. In the situation in which the operating surgeon is unable to obtain a 1-cm distal margin,[34] the slimmest acceptable margin, an APR is considered. In addition to this scenario, preoperative factors that point toward a benefit to APR include patient preference, poor preoperative continence, and/or tumors that obviously grow into the anal sphincter mechanism.[35] It is clear that a patient with preexisting fecal incontinence or sphincter injury has better function following an APR or other procedure with permanent colostomy than by the heroic attempt to save the anal sphincter and reestablish intestinal continuity. The technical details of APR are beyond the scope of this article, but it should be understood that one should avoid the waist observed in APR specimens, that is, a narrowing of the specimen that occurs as the dissection proceeds from superiorly into the levator hiatus. Unlike the original description of APRs in which the levator was transected off the lateral pelvic side wall, present techniques have evolved toward a closer dissection to the rectum at the proximal anal canal. This represents a potentially compromised radial margin at that point and probably explains the observed higher incidence of local failure after APR.[36,37]

ALGORITHM

The dissection for mid to low tumors of the rectum is conducted with standard TME techniques unless the tumor extends into adjoining structures and a negative circumferential margin is unobtainable. A standard proctectomy is performed, with an emphasis on complete extirpation of the mesorectal fascia and all of its contents, with nerve-sparing techniques and an aim toward obtaining negative margins. The technique is altered in the anterior plane, taking Denonvilliers' fascia with anterior or circumferential tumors and leaving this fascia with more posterior tumors for the sake of nerve preservation. As the dissection proceeds toward the anus, it is the authors' practice to frequently reassess margin status from the abdominal side and the transanal side. A distal margin of 1 cm for distal tumors is sufficient, as detailed earlier. At the level of the rectal lesion, the approach is to assure a negative circumferential margin. If the lesion appears to invade the pelvic floor and/or sphincter mechanism, the authors would elect to perform APR. If a 1-cm distal margin is unobtainable but circumferential margins appear clean, the authors' approach is to consider mucosectomy with hand-sewn anastomosis of one of the pelvic pouches described earlier. In this situation, the patient is warned of the functional consequences and a frozen section of the distal margin is obtained to rule out malignancy. A positive margin would necessitate APR.

OUTCOMES OF PROCTECTOMY FOR RECTAL CANCER

In addition to the more traditional outcomes of morbidity and mortality, oncologic, functional, and quality of life outcomes have undergone more thoughtful investigation in the recent past. Many surgical reports of outcomes following proctectomy have revealed high rates of morbidity and appreciable mortality. Unfortunately, the vast majority of those reports come from specialty centers with considerable experience in LAR techniques. Population-based rates of morbidity and mortality are difficult to obtain; however, a review from the National Surgical Quality Improvement Project revealed complications in 30% of patients after proctectomy and a 30-day mortality rate of 3.2% at Veterans Hospitals.[38] In addition, a 5% mortality was recorded after proctectomy in non–National Cancer Institute designated hospitals in the Survival, Epidemiology, and End Results—Medicare database.[39] These results reveal high rates of morbidity and mortality for proctectomy as compared with other abdominal or pelvic surgical procedures.

Oncologic results have been intensely scrutinized. Following LAR, oncologic results have been improving with the dispersion of the technique of TME. In contrast to LAR, patients who undergo curative-intent APR have significantly higher rates of bowel perforation, greater incidence of involved margins, and increased local recurrence, even after adjusting for tumor stage and size.[36,40,41] Although most experts claim that much of the increased difference in cancer recurrence with APR can be accounted for by the very aggressive biology of very low cancers,[42,43] there is an increased understanding that many of the difficulties encountered with APR outcomes are secondary to anatomic and technical issues that previously received minimal consideration. As described earlier, carrying the dissection along the mesorectal plane at the level of the pelvic floor may leave tumor behind when the rectal cancer invades the levator muscles.[44] An anatomic waist in the APR specimen is often seen with this method of coning at the levators. This phenomenon has been reinforced by a recent review, revealing little to no levator muscle excision in the proctectomy specimens of patients with rectal cancer.[36] Ultimately, oncologic outcomes are best when all resection margins are clean regardless of the procedure performed.

A growing area of interest in sphincter-sparing surgery is the understanding of functional outcomes following proctectomy. Bowel function or dysfunction is related to (1) the structural integrity and function of the pelvic floor, (2) the use of neoadjuvant or adjuvant radiotherapy, (3) the anastomotic level, and (4) the method of anastomotic reconstruction. In a follow-up to the Dutch TME trial,[45] 38.8% of nonirradiated and 61.5% of irradiated patients experienced fecal incontinence. Presumably, incontinence is worsened with removal of the internal sphincter or during mucosectomy. In addition to bowel dysfunction, pelvic dissection is associated with a risk of sexual or urinary dysfunction caused by autonomic nerve injury. Recent data from the Dutch TME trial suggest that approximately 75% of men and 60% of women suffer from sexual dysfunction following proctectomy.[46] Similarly, 38.1% of patients complained of urinary incontinence and 30.6% complained of impaired bladder emptying.[47]

Quality of life is also an important consideration when addressing outcomes following proctectomy. Data reveal an association between bowel function and overall quality of life. This is particularly true following the loss of fecal continence with APR, which leads to substantial reductions in quality of life.[48–50] Patients treated with APR are more likely to experience psychological distress, impaired social functioning, and greater sexual dysfunction.[48] However, others have demonstrated similar quality of life scores in patients with a stoma as compared with those patients who have undergone a restorative procedure. Although the outcomes data and information regarding patient preferences are critical, it should also be understood that a well-functioning stoma is better tolerated than a poorly functioning restorative procedure.

SUMMARY

Data reveal increasing adoption of LAR techniques over the past 2 decades. In this article, the authors have detailed the technical steps to preserve the anal sphincter and have outlined methods to optimize functional outcomes in the setting of low pelvic anastomosis for patients with rectal cancer. Surgery for rectal cancer, particularly those tumors of the distal rectum, remains challenging despite the numerous technical modifications aimed at sparing gastrointestinal continuity and improving outcomes.

REFERENCES

1. Delaney CP, MacKeigan JM. Preoperative management–risk assessment, medical evaluation, and bowel preparation. In: Wolff BG, Fleshman JW, Beck DE, et al, editors. The ASCRS textbook of colon and rectal surgery. New York: Springer Science+Business Media, LLC; 2007. p. 116.
2. Beets-Tan RG, Vliegen RF, Beets GL. Magnetic resonance imaging of rectal cancer: what radiation oncologists need to know. Front Radiat Ther Oncol 2004;38:1–12.
3. Brown G, Davies S, Williams GT, et al. Effectiveness of preoperative staging in rectal cancer: digital rectal examination, endoluminal ultrasound or magnetic resonance imaging? Br J Cancer 2004;91(1):23–9.
4. Brown G, Daniels IR. Preoperative staging of rectal cancer: the MERCURY research project. Recent Results Cancer Res 2005;165:58–74.
5. Brown G. Thin section MRI in multidisciplinary pre-operative decision making for patients with rectal cancer. Br J Radiol 2005;78(Spec No 2):S117–27.
6. Sauer R, Becker H, Hohenberger W, et al. Preoperative versus postoperative chemoradiotherapy for rectal cancer. N Engl J Med 2004;351(17):1731–40.

7. The National Comprehensive Cancer Network. Rectal cancer clinical practice guidelines in oncology. J Natl Compr Canc Netw 2005;3(4):492–508.
8. Heald RJ. A new approach to rectal cancer. Br J Hosp Med 1979;22(3):277–81.
9. Heald RJ, Husband EM, Ryall RD. The mesorectum in rectal cancer surgery-the clue to pelvic recurrence? Br J Surg 1982;69(10):613–6.
10. Quirke P, Durdey P, Dixon MF, et al. Local recurrence of rectal adenocarcinoma due to inadequate surgical resection. Histopathological study of lateral tumour spread and surgical excision. Lancet 1986;2(8514):996–9.
11. Adam IJ, Mohamdee MO, Martin IG, et al. Role of circumferential margin involvement in the local recurrence of rectal cancer. Lancet 1994;344(8924): 707–11.
12. Nagtegaal ID, Marijnen CA, Kranenbarg EK, et al. Circumferential margin involvement is still an important predictor of local recurrence in rectal carcinoma: not one millimeter but two millimeters is the limit. Am J Surg Pathol 2002;26(3):350–7.
13. Wibe A, Rendedal PR, Svensson E, et al. Prognostic significance of the circumferential resection margin following total mesorectal excision for rectal cancer. Br J Surg 2002;89(3):327–34.
14. Martling AL, Holm T, Rutqvist LE, et al. Effect of a surgical training programme on outcome of rectal cancer in the County of Stockholm. Stockholm Colorectal Cancer Study Group, Basingstoke Bowel Cancer Research Project. Lancet 2000;356(9224):93–6.
15. Williams NS. The rationale for preservation of the anal sphincter in patients with low rectal cancer. Br J Surg 1984;71(8):575–81.
16. Schiessel R, Novi G, Holzer B, et al. Technique and long-term results of intersphincteric resection for low rectal cancer. Dis Colon Rectum 2005;48(10):1858–67.
17. Parks AG, Percy JP. Resection and sutured colo-anal anastomosis for rectal carcinoma. Br J Surg 1982;69(6):301–14.
18. Baker JW. Low end to side rectosigmoidal anastomosis; description of technique. Arch Surg 1950;61(1):143–57.
19. Lazorthes F, Fages P, Chiotasso P, et al. Resection of the rectum with construction of a colonic reservoir and colo-anal anastomosis for carcinoma of the rectum. Br J Surg 1986;73(2):136–8.
20. Parc R, Tiret E, Frileux P, et al. Resection and colo-anal anastomosis with colonic reservoir for rectal carcinoma. Br J Surg 1986;73(2):139–41.
21. Willis S, Hölzl F, Wein B. The functional principle of the colonic J-pouch is not its reservoir function but a delay of colonic motility. Int J Colorectal Dis 2007;22(2): 161–5.
22. Lazorthes F, Gamagami R, Chiotasso P, et al. Prospective randomized study comparing clinical results between small and large colonic J-pouch following coloanal anastomosis. Dis Colon Rectum 1997;40(12):1409–13.
23. Harris GJC, Lavery IJ, Fazio VW. Reasons for failure to construct to colonic J pouch. What can be done to improve the size of the neorectal reservoir should it occur? Dis Colon Rectum 2002;45(10):1304–8.
24. Hida J, Yasutomi M, Maruyama T, et al. Indications for colonic J pouch reconstruction after anterior resection for rectal cancer: determining the optimal level of anastomosis. Dis Colon Rectum 1998;41(5):558–63.
25. Sailer M, Fuchs HK, Fein M, et al. Randomized clinical trial comparing quality of life after straight and pouch coloanal reconstruction. Br J Surg 2002;89(9):1108–17.
26. Ho YH, Brown S, Heah SM, et al. Comparison of J-pouch and coloplasty pouch for low rectal cancers. Ann Surg 2002;236(1):49–55.

27. Fazio VW, Zutshi M, Remzi FH, et al. A randomized multicenter trial to compare long-term functional outcome, quality of life, and complications of surgical procedures for low rectal cancers. Ann Surg 2007;246(3):481–8.

28. Machado M, Nygren J, Goldman S, et al. Similar outcome after colonic pouch and side-to-end anastomosis in low anterior resection for rectal cancer: a prospective randomized trial. Ann Surg 2003;238(2):214–20.

29. Brown CJ. Reconstructive techniques after rectal resection for rectal cancer. Cochrane Database Syst Rev 2008;2:CD006040.

30. Dehni N, Schlegel RD, Cunningham C, et al. Influence of a defunctioning stoma on leakage rates after low colorectal anastomosis and colonic J pouch-anal anastomosis. Br J Surg 1998;85(8):1114–7.

31. Marusch F, Koch A, Schmidt HD, et al. Value of protective stoma in low anterior resections for rectal carcinoma. Dis Colon Rectum 2002;45(9):1164–71.

32. Tan WS, Tang CL, Shi L, et al. Meta-analysis of defunctioning stomas in low anterior resection for rectal cancer. Br J Surg 2009;96(5):462–72.

33. Hüser N, Michalski CW, Erkan M, et al. Systematic review and meta-analysis of the role of defunctioning stoma in low rectal cancer surgery. Ann Surg 2008; 248(1):52–60.

34. Vernava AM, Moran M. A prospective evaluation of distal margins in carcinoma of the rectum. Surg Gynecol Obstet 1992;175(4):333–6.

35. Wolmark N, Wieand HS, Hyams DM, et al. Randomized trial of postoperative adjuvant chemotherapy with or without radiotherapy for carcinoma of the rectum. National Surgical Adjuvant Breast and Bowel Project, protocol R-02. J Natl Cancer Inst 2000;92(5):388–96.

36. Nagtegaal ID, van de Velde CJ, Marijnen CA, et al. Low rectal cancer: a call for a change of approach in abdominoperineal resection. J Clin Oncol 2005;23(36): 9257–64.

37. Marr R, Birbeck K, Garcivan J, et al. The Modern Abdominoperineal Excision. The next challenge after total mesorectal excision. Ann Surg 2005;242(1):74–82.

38. Longo WE, Virgo KS, Johnson FE, et al. Outcome after proctectomy for rectal cancer in Department of Veterans Affairs Hospitals: a report from the National Surgical Quality Improvement Program. Ann Surg 1998;228(1):64–70.

39. Paulson EC, Mitra N, Sonnad S, et al. National Cancer Institute designation predicts improved outcomes in colorectal cancer surgery. Ann Surg 2008; 248(4):675–86.

40. Daniels I. MRI predicts surgical resection margin status in patients with rectal cancer: results from the MERCURY Study Group. Clin Oncol 2004;16:S45–6.

41. Eriksen MT, Wibe A, Syse A, et al. Inadvertent perforation during rectal cancer resection in Norway. Br J Surg 2004;91(2):210–6.

42. Hojo K, Koyama Y. Lymphatic spread and its prognostic value in patients with rectal cancer. Am J Surg 1982;144(3):350–4.

43. Hermanek P. Current aspects of a new staging classification of colorectal cancer and its clinical consequences. Chirurg 1989;60(1):1–7.

44. Salerno G, Chandler I, Wotherspoon A, et al. Sites of surgical wasting in the abdominoperineal specimen. Br J Surg 2008;95(9):1147–54.

45. Lange MM, den Dulk M, Bossema ER, et al. Risk factors for faecal incontinence after rectal cancer treatment. Br J Surg 2007;94(10):1278–84.

46. Lange MM, Marijnen CA, Maas CP, et al. Risk factors for sexual dysfunction after rectal cancer treatment. Eur J Cancer 2009;45(9):1578–88.

47. Lange MM, Maas CP, Marijnen CA, et al. Urinary dysfunction after rectal cancer treatment is mainly caused by surgery. Br J Surg 2008;95(8):1020–8.

48. Sprangers MA, Taal BG, Aaronson NK, et al. Quality of life in colorectal cancer. Stoma vs. nonstoma patients. Dis Colon Rectum 1995;38(4):361–9.
49. Camilleri-Brennan J, Steele RJ. Quality of life after treatment for rectal cancer. Br J Surg 1998;85(8):1036–43.
50. Williams NS, Johnston D. The quality of life after rectal excision for low rectal cancer. Br J Surg 1983;70(8):460–2.

Laparoscopy for Colon Cancer: State of the Art

Gaetano Luglio, MD[a], Heidi Nelson, MD[b],*

KEYWORDS

• Laparoscopy • Colon • Cancer • Colectomy

Minimally invasive surgery has rapidly evolved in the past 2 decades, revolutionizing surgical practice such that laparoscopic techniques are now favored for common abdominal procedures. The same has been true for laparoscopic colectomy, with the exception of the indication of colon cancer. When laparoscopic surgery was first considered in the early 1990s, several oncologic concerns were raised. Early reports of wound tumor implants raised the question of whether it was appropriate to implement laparoscopic techniques, particularly pneumoperitoneum, in cases in which a patient has potentially curable disease. Additional questions regarded the adequacy of laparoscopic surgery in achieving a proper oncologic resection, in particular, lymph node harvest, exploration of the abdomen, and general staging. Little was known about whether laparoscopy would alter the patterns of tumor cell dissemination.

Despite these concerns, patients expressed strong interest in this new, minimally invasive approach to colon resection. The possibility of benefits continued to drive laparoscopic surgery into surgical oncology. After several years of study, the risk/benefit discussion can be finalized with respect to laparoscopic colectomy for curable cancer. This article discusses results from several large, international, prospective, randomized trials addressing 3 key questions. First, why have thousands of patients accepted participation in a laparoscopic trial knowing that they might have an inferior oncologic result? Second, what oncologic lessons have been learned from so many years of clinical trials? And third, what are the current technical approaches that are in use, and what does the future hold for new advances in robotics and natural-orifice surgery?

WHY HAVE PATIENTS PARTICIPATED IN LAPAROSCOPIC COLECTOMY TRIALS?

Most patients, and many physicians, assumed that laparoscopic colectomy would offer advantages in recovery similar to those experienced for laparoscopic

[a] Department of General, Oncological and Minimally-Invasive Surgery - Surgical Coloproctology Unit, Federico II University, Via Pansini 5, 80131 Naples, Italy
[b] Division of Colon and Rectal Surgery, Department of Surgery, Mayo Clinic, 200 First Street SW, Gonda 9-205, Rochester, MN 55905, USA
* Corresponding author.
E-mail address: nelson.heidi@mayo.edu

Surg Oncol Clin N Am 19 (2010) 777–791
doi:10.1016/j.soc.2010.07.003   surgonc.theclinics.com

cholecystectomy. However, it took several years and many carefully conducted clinical trials to precisely define the degree of benefit. Because the oncologic issues were perceived as representing a potential threat to the oncologic outcomes of these patients, several prospective, randomized trials were designed to examine the benefits in the context of the risks. The field had reached a point of equipoise at which the patients and many surgeons preferred the laparoscopic approach, whereas the oncologic risks were uncertain and unknown. This formed the basis of several international clinical trials, as described later. Each of the trials was designed to rigorously investigate the feasibility of laparoscopic colectomy and the cancer risk and recovery benefits in the setting of curable colon cancer.

At least 4 large, prospective, randomized controlled trials from North America, Canada, and Europe have been completed and have reported both short- and long-term outcomes. To date, 3133 patients have been studied by random allocation to laparoscopic versus open surgery and followed for cancer and short-term outcomes. These patients are reported from the Barcelona Trial (219 patients),[1,2] the Clinical Outcomes of Surgical Therapy (COST) Trial (872 patients),[3,4] the Colon Cancer Laparoscopic or Open Resection (COLOR) Trial (1248 patients),[5,6] and the Conventional versus Laparoscopic-Assisted Surgery in Patients with Colorectal Cancer (CLASSIC) Trial (794 patients)[7,8]; the novel aspect of the CLASSIC trial is its inclusion of patients with rectal cancer.

POTENTIAL BENEFITS AND SHORT-TERM OUTCOMES

Why have thousands of patients accepted participation in laparoscopic trials knowing that they might have an inferior oncologic result?

The driver of laparoscopic colectomy in the setting of cancer was the possibility of gaining patient benefits. It was presumed, but not proved, that a shorter incision would result in less pain, short-duration ileus, and shorter hospital and posthospitalization recovery. To measure these potential benefits, several metrics were developed. Most of the clinical trials measured end points such as length of incision, duration of ileus, the need for analgesia, duration of hospital stay, quality of life (QOL), and complications. Such measurements try to capture the full patient experience, from physiologic factors to the patient's perception of recovery. In 1993, when many of the international trials were launched, these tools were neither widely accepted nor well developed. Nevertheless, it was possible to identify patient-related benefits, as discussed later.

Data on recovery end points are available, showing the main advantages of the laparoscopic approach: length of hospital stay, duration of ileus, and duration of analgesic use or postoperative pain (**Table 1**). The COLOR, CLASSIC, and Barcelona trials have found a shorter postoperative ileus with an earlier resumption of fluid intake and a normal diet in the laparoscopic arm. The COST trial showed a significant reduction in duration of narcotic and oral analgesic requirement, and the COLOR trial has shown a lower need for opioid analgesics on postoperative day 2 and 3 in the laparoscopic arm.

Another more recent single-institution, controlled trial from Taiwan[9] randomized 286 patients with more selective entry criteria, including only tumors located in the distal transverse and left colon, requiring mobilization of the splenic flexure. The Taiwan trial is the only one to compare postoperative pain using a visual analog scale, underlying how laparoscopic surgery allows better pain control. Data on postoperative pain control are also available from other studies; in a review article, Tjandra and Chan[10] showed that 7 randomized studies reported significantly less pain, by 12.6%, after

Table 1
Laparoscopic-assisted colectomy (LAC) versus open colectomy (OC): recovery benefits

	Hospital Stay (d) LAC vs OC	Duration of Ileus LAC vs OC	Duration of Analgesics (d) LAC vs OC
COST	5 vs 6 ($P<.001$)	—	Oral, 1 vs 2 ($P = 0.002$) Intravenous, 3 vs 4 ($P<.001$)
COLOR	8.2 vs 9.3 ($P<.0001$)	3.6 vs 4.6 (days to BM) ($P<.0001$)	—
CLASSIC	9 vs 11	5 vs 6 (days to BM)	—
Barcelona	5.2 vs 7.9 ($P = .005$)	36 vs 55 (hours to peristalsis) ($P<.001$)	—

Abbreviations: BM, bowel movements; d, days.

laparoscopic procedures, as shown by a reduction of several pain scores, together with a reduction of 30.7% in the use of postoperative narcotics. A Cochrane Database review,[11] based on results from 6 trials, also showed significantly reduced postoperative pain perception on the first postoperative day; however, no significant differences in pain perception were assessed on the second postoperative day.

Data available from the Taiwan trial also demonstrate how laparoscopic surgery–related benefits go beyond enhanced hospital parameters because of better postoperative and posthospital recovery, with a significantly shorter return to partial activity, full activity, and ordinary work.

Intraoperative outcomes were also addressed, showing additional benefits gained through the use of laparoscopic techniques (**Table 2**). The length of incision was significantly shorter in laparoscopic arms. Investigators from the Taiwan trial argued that, even if open colectomies could be performed in thinner patients through a small incision (<7 cm), the benefits of laparoscopic surgery go beyond the wound size, because there are recovery advantages, a magnified operative field, and a more precise resection of the tumor.

Recovery benefits are gained at the expense of a longer duration of surgery for those treated with laparoscopic colectomy. The duration of surgery in the laparoscopic arm in each of the trials ranged from 24 to 55 minutes more than the open arm, and this difference was significant. Laparoscopic surgery is more costly. The Taiwan trial reported that the overall cost of laparoscopic procedures is significantly higher. However, multicenter randomized data on the costs of the laparoscopic approach are poor. Results are variable on costs, with some studies showing higher overall costs, mostly because of the use of disposable instruments and longer operative times. Other studies show cost saving because of reduced length of hospital stay. Costs seem to be highly practice dependent.

Table 2
LAC versus OC: intraoperative outcomes

	Operative Time (min) LAC vs OC	Blood Loss (mL) LAC vs OC	Length of Incision (cm) LAC vs OC
COST	150 vs 95 ($P<.001$)	—	18 vs 6 ($P<.001$)
COLOR	145 vs 115 ($P<.001$)	100 vs 175 ($P<.003$)	—
CLASSIC	180 vs 135	—	10 vs 22
Barcelona	142 vs 118 ($P<.001$)	105 vs 193 ($P<.001$)	4.5 (left), 6.5 (right)

Short-term complications, morbidity, and mortality were investigated and found to be similar between groups in all the trials (**Table 3**). Thirty-day mortality was not significantly different among trials, although the CLASSIC trial reported higher mortality in both the laparoscopic and open arm compared with the other studies. No significant differences in the rates of intraoperative complications, rates and severity of postoperative complications at discharge, and rates of readmission or reoperation were identified by any of the biggest multicenter randomized trials. However, the Barcelona Trial reported a significant reduction in postoperative complication in the laparoscopic arm.

Other than the main trials mentioned earlier, several studies report on short-term outcomes and morbidity after laparoscopic and open colectomy for colon cancer. One of the most remarkable was led by Bilimoria and colleagues,[12] in which data available from 3059 patients from 121 hospitals were analyzed, using the American College of Surgeons National Surgical Quality Improvement Project database. Although no differences were found in mortality and reoperation rate, the laparoscopic colectomy group showed a significantly lower overall morbidity, attributed to better outcomes for surgical site infections and pneumonia. A significantly lower rate of wound complications (combining wound infection and wound dehiscence) after laparoscopic colectomy was also shown in the pooled analysis of 17 randomized, controlled trials on laparoscopic resection for colon cancer by Tjandra and Chan,[10] although no significant differences in overall complication rates were found between the 2 arms.

Although these findings are likely explained by selection bias, it is also possible that there is some additional benefit to laparoscopic surgery from either the lesser extent of wounding or the better preservation of the immune status.

QOL

Regarding QOL parameters, there is now substantial evidence to support modest QOL benefits for patients who have cancer treated with laparoscopic colectomy. The meta-analysis from the Cochrane Database on short-term outcomes after laparoscopic surgery[11] shows that there are only 2 randomized trials that have appropriately investigated QOL after laparoscopic and open colectomy for cancer. The pooled data from these 2 studies failed to show any significant advantage for the laparoscopic versus the conventional technique 60 days after surgery. The COST study, led by Weeks and Nelson,[13] investigated 428 patients, using 3 different QOL scores, evaluating outcomes at 2 days, 2 weeks, and 2 months after surgery. The only statistically significant difference between the 2 arms was identified at 2 weeks after surgery, showing a slightly better overall QOL.

It remains unclear why laparoscopic-assisted colectomy (LAC) has not shown QOL benefits as significant as other parameters of postoperative recovery. One possible explanation could arise from the high conversion rates: data were analyzed by

Table 3		
LAC versus OC: perioperative morbidity and mortality		
	Morbidity (%)	Mortality (%)
	LAC vs OC	LAC vs OC
COST	21 vs 20 ($P = 0.64$)	<1 vs 1 ($P = .40$)
COLOR	21 vs 20 ($P = .90$)	1 vs 2 ($P = .47$)
CLASSIC	35 vs 35 ($P = .78$)	4 vs 5
Barcelona	11 vs 29 ($P = .001$)	1 vs 3

intention-to-treat and this might have masked the favorable effect on QOL of cases that were completed laparoscopically, considering that converted cases were analyzed with the laparoscopic arm. Further gains in QOL in this situation would require substantial reductions in rates of conversion. Another possible explanation for the modest QOL benefits might derive from the inability of the currently available tools to appropriately measure QOL after laparoscopic surgery for carcinoma. Patients who have undergone surgery for carcinoma might evaluate their QOL differently from patients who underwent analogous surgery for benign disease, for which cosmesis, postoperative pain, and limitation of social activity might play a more relevant role.

Data from all relevant trials allow researchers to summarize the main patient-related benefits of the application of laparoscopic techniques in colon cancer resection. These benefits have been established by multicenter, randomized, controlled trials and meta-analysis, and level 1 evidence is now available to support them (see Ref.[14]):

1. General feasibility
2. Smaller incision
3. Lower narcotic usefulness
4. Reduced postoperative pain
5. Shorter hospitalization
6. Improved QOL (at 2 weeks after surgery)
7. Shorter postoperative recovery
8. Equivalent morbidity.

FUTURE DIRECTIONS FOR EVALUATING BENEFITS: LAPAROSCOPIC SURGERY IN THE ELDERLY

As mentioned earlier, patient-related benefits might be maximized by reducing rates of conversion; a reasonable goal regardless of the metric. Another possibility is to identify unique populations of patients who might achieve benefits beyond those achieved in the standard population. Aging patients may be among those unique subpopulations.

The risk of developing colon cancer increases with advancing age, with the median age at diagnosis reported as 71 years by United States National Cancer Institute (NCI) Surveillance, Epidemiology and End Results Program. Given that elderly patients are more susceptible to postoperative complications, such as cardiac and respiratory morbidities, they may do better with laparoscopic surgery than their younger counterparts. To explore this issue, some investigators have examined the effect of laparoscopic surgery on alterations in respiratory function and other physiologic parameters.[15] It seems that laparoscopic surgery may be associated with better respiratory function and other physiologic functions, supporting the possibility of better postoperative morbidity outcomes in the elderly.

Data available from trials also solve this issue for laparoscopic colectomy for cancer: a subset analysis from the COST trial shows that no differences in perioperative morbidity exist between open and laparoscopic groups in patients aged 70 years and older. In a previous matched-control study by Stocchi and Nelson,[16] 42 patients who underwent LAC and 42 patient who underwent open colectomy were compared; all the patients studied were older than 75 years with a high rate of patients who were American Society of Anesthesiologists (ASA) III and ASA IV (55% in the laparoscopic group and 64% in the open group). The investigators found that patients undergoing laparoscopic resection showed a reduction in morbidity, narcotic use, time to return to bowel movements, and length of hospital stay; the use of laparoscopic techniques not only reduced the length of hospital stay compared with open surgery, but this was reduced to nearly the same length of hospitalization for laparoscopic colectomies in the general population. This finding is important given the usual discrepancies between the elderly and general population in length of stay. The most relevant finding from this study is the preservation of postoperative independence in the laparoscopic group; it has been reported that only 67% of elderly patients return home after abdominal procedures,[17] whereas these data show that 95% of patients in the laparoscopic group remained independent after surgery. The most noteworthy finding from this report is that not only does laparoscopic surgery seem to give benefits in terms of morbidity, faster postoperative recovery, and preservation of functional status, but these benefits are even more remarkable in elderly patients than in the general population.

COLON CANCER AND LAPAROSCOPIC SURGERY: ONCOLOGIC LESSONS

As mentioned earlier, soon after the introduction of laparoscopic colectomy in 1991,[18] several concerns regarding the application of this technique in colon cancer were raised, such that national statements were issued recommending a moratorium on laparoscopic colectomy for cancer outside clinical trials.[19] One additional early concern regarding LAC for carcinoma was that laparoscopy would not allow adequate tactile sensation and might impair proper intraoperative tumor staging, especially with respect to evaluation of the liver. However, laparoscopic ultrasonography has been developed, both experimentally and clinically,[20,21] to improve accuracy in the intraoperative evaluation of the liver for metastatic disease. Furthermore, hand-assisted laparoscopic surgery (HALS) has been proposed as a variant of LAC that would allow resumption of complete tactile sensation.

ONCOLOGIC OUTCOMES

All the trials were able to demonstrate the noninferiority of laparoscopic surgery to open resection regarding oncologic outcomes. The most important end point that trials assessed was overall survival (**Table 4**). No significant differences were found in overall survival between the laparoscopic and open arm within each trial; however, results are different among trials considering, for example, that overall survival in open arms varies from 51% in the Barcelona Trial to 74.6% in the COST trial. Results regarding disease-free survival (DFS) also show no differences between open and laparoscopic arms in each trial, and these are shown in **Table 4**, together with results from a pooled analysis[22] of all 4 European and American trials; this meta-analysis

Table 4			
LAC versus OC: oncologic outcomes			
	Number of Patients	OS (%) LAC vs OC	DFS (%) LAC vs OC
COST (5 y)	872	76.4 vs 74.6 (P = .93)	69.2 vs 68.4 (P = .94)
COLOR (5 y)	1248	73.8 vs 74.2	66.5 vs 67.9
CLASSIC (3 y)	794	68.4 vs 66.7 (P = .51)	66.3 vs 67.7 (P = .75)
Barcelona (5 y)	219	64 vs 51 (P = .06)	—
Meta-analysis[a] (3 y)	1536	75.8 vs 75.3 (P = .92)	82.2 vs 83.5 (P = .61)

Abbreviations: DFS, disease-free survival; OS, overall survival.
[a] Transatlantic Laparoscopically Assisted versus Open Colectomy Trials Study Group.

examines the 3-year median oncologic outcomes from trials, reassuring the oncologic feasibility and safety of LAC for cancer with the following results: DFS rates in the laparoscopically assisted and open arms were 75.8% and 75.3% respectively; overall survival was 82.2% after laparoscopic surgery and 83.5% after open surgery; the meta-analysis showed no differences in oncologic outcomes for stage I, II, and III colon cancer between the 2 treatments.

The major trials also addressed the issue of recurrence rates between open and laparoscopic groups for other oncologic end points. Overall recurrence, local recurrence, and wound recurrence rates are shown in **Table 5**, together with the extend follow-up. No significant differences were found between the 2 arms of each trial, although, as mentioned earlier, different results were achieved in local and overall recurrence among trials.

No differences existed in wound recurrence rates between laparoscopic and open arms; this finding seems particularly significant because laparoscopic surgery for colon cancer was controversial at first, causing some reports to present alarming incidences of port-site recurrences. Investigators from the Taiwan trial focused on recurrence rates and time to recurrence; besides an equivalent time to recurrence, this trial showed a similar recurrence pattern between the 2 arms, and, although the possibility of port-site recurrences is confirmed, the risk seems to be low and, when laparoscopic procedures are performed according to strict oncologic principles, the risk of intraperitoneal cancer spillage is not increased.

These results show that level 1 evidence is now available to support the advantages, and to refute the disadvantages, of laparoscopic colectomy in curable colon cancer. The COST investigators showed that these finding were consistent in all stages of disease and persistent in multivariant analysis, adjusting for stratification factors. Trials have demonstrated that, even if measures that are surrogate markers of a correct oncological resection (proximal/distal margin, length of mesentery and number of lymph nodes) are considered, LAC is no longer inferior to its open counterpart. The meta-analysis[22] also shows the comparison of the number of lymph nodes harvested during surgery: the mean ($\pm$SD) number of lymph nodes found in the laparoscopically resected specimens was 11.8 ($\pm$7.4), whereas 12.2 ($\pm$7.8) lymph nodes were found in the specimens obtained in open colectomy; analysis of variance showed that this was not statistically different and that the difference did not statistically vary among the 4 studies.

In 2002, Lacy and colleagues[1] reported improved survival after laparoscopic colectomy in patients with stage III colon cancer, and this result was confirmed in 2008.[2] However, the outcome of this study was called into question because the total number of patients was low, the study involved a single laparoscopic center, and there were concerns about the results being limited to a small subset of patients with stage III

Table 5
LAC versus OC: overall recurrence (OR), local recurrence (LR), wound recurrence (WR)

	OR (%)	LR (%)	WR (%)
	LAC vs OC	LAC vs OC	LAC vs OC
COST (5 y)	19.4 vs 21.8 ($P = .25$)	2.3 vs 2.6 ($P = .79$)	0.9 vs 0.5 ($P = .43$)
COLOR (5 y)	19.6 vs 16.9 ($P = .24$)	9.1 vs 7 ($P = .24$)	1.3 vs 0.4 ($P = .09$)
CLASSIC (3 y)	23.8 vs 22.2 ($P = .74$)	8.6 vs 7.9 ($P = .76$)	2.5 vs 0.6 ($P = .12$)
Barcelona (5 y)	18 vs 28 ($P = .07$)	7.5 vs 13.7 ($P = .65$)	0.9 vs 0 ($P = .65$)

disease. Most of the studies, including the United States prospective multicenter randomized trial, have not been able to reproduce the findings of the trial by Lacy and colleagues,[1] even when stage-specific comparisons were undertaken.

CURRENT TECHNICAL APPROACHES: MEDIAL-TO-LATERAL, LATERAL-TO-MEDIAL, AND HAND-ASSISTED SURGERY
Medial-to-lateral and Lateral-to-medial Approaches

Both right and left colectomies can be performed using 2 main approaches: lateral to medial or medial to lateral. The lateral-to-medial approach is based on a dissection sequence similar to that of conventional open surgery. For example, with the right colectomy, after trocar placement and abdominal exploration, the peritoneum around the base of the terminal ileum and the cecum is incised and the correct retroperitoneal plane is entered. The ureter is identified either before opening the peritoneum in a thin patient or after the peritoneum is incised. Using a grasper on the cut peritoneal edge, the right lateral peritoneal reflection is opened along the white line of Toldt toward the hepatic flexure. As the dissection proceeds toward the hepatic flexure, the retroperitoneal planes are developed, with care being taken to identify and protect the duodenum. The plane of retroperitoneal dissection is just beneath the colon mesentery, which ensures that the dissection will be above the plane of Gerota fascia and away from the kidney. The peritoneum on the medial side of the terminal ileum should be incised to allow full mobilization of the cecum; the dissection is continued up to the level of the duodenum. Then the lateral dissection is advanced medially with care until the inferior vena cava inferiorly and duodenum superiorly; these 2 structures indicate the achievement of sufficient medial dissection.

The left hemicolectomy procedure is similar to the right colectomy, only in mirror-image reverse. One major difference is the care that must be taken around the spleen.

The medial-to-lateral approach is an alternative technique for both right and left colectomy; in this case the mesocolon is dissected starting from the medial side, identifying and ligating the vessels at their origin. The retroperitoneum is entered, and blunt and cautery dissection allows the colon to be freed from the peritoneal attachments on the medial side; the dissection continues along the white line of Toldt so that the colon is detached from all the attachments.

Vascular ligation and anastomosis can be performed either by incorporeal or extracorporeal methods. No additional patient benefits have been demonstrated for the complete intracorporeal approach, and a small incision is required to extract the specimen.[23]

The choice between the lateral-to-medial or medial-to-lateral techniques is a matter of preference and training, and there is no evidence favoring the use of either approach. Some studies[24,25] comparing the 2 techniques favor the medial approach because of a supposed shorter operative time, but they failed to demonstrate any advantages in postoperative recovery parameters, complications, or oncologic outcomes. Whichever approach is preferred, a few key principles should be followed.[26] These principles include making the procedure as simple as possible, reproducible, easy to teach, and easy to learn; this is achieved by making the laparoscopic procedure as close to the open procedure as possible and for this reason the lateral approach could be preferred.

HAND-ASSISTED COLECTOMY

Despite trials showing the noninferiority of the laparoscopic approach in colon cancer treatment, and despite the indisputable short-term patient-related benefits, with equal disease-specific outcomes and improved recovery profile, minimally invasive surgery for colonic diseases is not yet widespread; according to the results of some studies,[27,28] only 3% to 8% of colectomies performed annually in the United States use true laparoscopic techniques. The main reason for this situation is that laparoscopic colectomy is not easy to perform; surgeons are obliged to operate in multiple abdominal quadrants on a mobile organ, so they have to be proficient at laparoscopic surgery to take on laparoscopic colectomy.

HALS has emerged as a kind of bridge between open and laparoscopic colectomy. This technique allows the surgeon to put a hand inside the abdomen, permitting palpation, retraction, and blunt dissection, along with easier bleeding control. The main tool is a special hand-access device that allows maintenance of pneumoperitoneum while the surgeon's hand is inside the abdomen. At the same time, the hand-port incision (6–7 cm) allows the extraction of the specimen. The hand-assisted colectomy can be performed following all the oncologic resection principles as well as the laparoscopic approach.

The Mayo Clinic experience shows remarkable results with hand-assisted colectomy in a study population of 969 patients (373 HALS and 596 LAC)[29]; these results are shown in **Table 6** and show a reduction in operating time and conversion rate with the same complication rate; the average hospital stay is 1 day longer in the HALS group, but this seems to be caused by more complex cases being approached with the HALS technique. This study therefore shows that HALS could become the preferred technique to perform more challenging procedures (such as left colectomy, low anterior resection, and total colectomy), allowing the expansion of minimally invasive practice to patients who otherwise might not have been considered candidates for laparoscopic surgery. At the same time, HALS may be a useful tool for shortening the learning process associated with performing laparoscopic colectomy.

Another single-institution experience with hand-assisted surgery comes from the Cleveland Clinic,[30] which report similar results between laparoscopic and hand-assisted groups in short-term outcomes such as operative time, conversion rates, length of hospital stay, and overall morbidity. This study also focused on costs associated with the HALS procedure, which is important considering recent concerns about the costs of surgical practice; median total cost seems not to be statistically different between the 2 groups; the operating room costs are increased in the HALS

Table 6
LAC versus hand-assisted laparoscopic colectomy (HALC): short-term outcomes

	Conversion Rate (%)	Operating Time (min)	Overall Morbidity (%)	Length of Stay (d)	Total Cost (US$)
	LAC vs HALC	LAC vs HALC	LAC vs HALC	LAC vs HALC	LAC vs HALC
Mayo Clinic (969 patients)	15.3 vs 3.4 (*P*<.001)	258 ± 90 vs 242 ± 89 (*P* = .037)	13.6 vs 15.4 (*P* = .629)	5 ± 3 vs 6 ± 3.4 (*P*<.001)	—
Cleveland Clinic (200 patients)	4 vs 3 (*P* = 1)	163 ± 65 vs 168 ± 61 (*P* = .57)	32 vs 16 (*P* = .009)	4(3–7) vs 4(3–6) (*P* = .58)	8373 vs 8521 (*P* = .79)
US multicenter, randomized, controlled trial (95 patients) (Marcello et al[31])	12.5 vs 2 (*P* = .11)	285 ± 105 vs 199 ± 35 (*P* = .015)	19 vs 21 (*P* = .68)	8.9 ± 11.5 vs 6.9 ± 8 (*P* = .58) for total colectomy	—

group, but total cost tends to be similar, perhaps because of higher consultation and emergency services in the LAC group. These results are shown in **Table 6**, and are compared with Mayo Clinic outcomes and with results from another United States multicenter randomized trial,[31] focusing in particular on a significantly shorter operative time achieved through hand-assisted colectomy while maintaining similar short-term outcomes such as overall complication rate, time to return to bowel function, tolerance of diet, postoperative pain, narcotic usage, and length of hospitalization.

Despite these data showing the advantages of the hand-assisted approach, it could be argued that, in most cases, the hand-assisted technique requires a significantly larger incision, and this might be concerning in laparoscopic surgery because cosmesis plays an important role. This technique could represent a drawback regarding the improvement of laparoscopic skills, arresting the learning process, rather than working as a bridge; it could represent a backward step, requiring the surgeon to put a hand in the patient's abdomen again. Probably the best way to consider this more recent approach is not to consider it as a replacement to total laparoscopic surgery, but as one more tool in the surgeon's armamentarium that can be used if it is required.

CURRENT INDICATIONS AND CONTRAINDICATIONS

Considering all the data and results supporting the safety of the laparoscopic approach in colon cancer surgery, contraindications for laparoscopic colon cancer resection are the same as for laparoscopic surgery in general.

General health conditions that would contraindicate a minimally invasive approach requiring a pneumoperitoneum typically include any severe manifestation of organ failure, such as severe chronic obstructive pulmonary disease or other causes of respiratory compromise, advanced cardiovascular diseases, end-organ renal failure, and severe electrolyte or fluid disturbances, and patients with liver failure, ascites, or other sources of bleeding disorders are best served with a more controlled, open approach. Less-absolute or relative contraindications of laparoscopy include the presence of adhesions, cardiac abnormalities, pulmonary gas exchange abnormalities, chronic liver disease, and obesity. None of these are absolute. For example, patients may have several abdominal scars and may have undergone numerous prior procedures, even near the site of the anticipated colon resection, but they may not have prohibitive adhesions. Unless the patient has prohibitive adhesions, we would approach the case laparoscopically, with a cautionary note to the patient that the risk of conversion may be higher than 10% to 15%. The same can be said for obesity. Sometimes, managing obese patients is facilitated by laparoscopy, such as when the fat is predominantly in the abdominal wall. However, obesity cases cannot be conducted using laparoscopic technique if the tools do not reach from the port to the site of the surgical resection.

Regarding cancer specific issues, there is little evidence in support of tackling large, fixed, or recurrent tumors through small incisions. The risk/benefit ratio for large, fixed, and recurrent tumors would likely favor open surgery, although this has never been prospectively studied. Based on these findings, the National Comprehensive Cancer Network (NCCN) wrote guidelines for 2010, stating that LAC for cancer may be considered using the following criteria:

- Surgeon with experience performing laparoscopically assisted colorectal surgery
- No disease in rectum or prohibitive abdominal adhesion

- No locally advanced disease
- Not indicated for acute small bowel obstruction or perforation from cancer
- Thorough abdominal exploration is required
- Consider preoperative marking of small lesion.

According to NCCN guidelines, all other oncologic principles for colon cancer operations should also be addressed in laparoscopic-assisted surgery, particularly regarding lymph node harvesting: nodes at the origin of a feeding vessel should be identified for pathologic examination and a minimum of 12 lymph nodes is necessary to establish N stage.

To date, not all the findings regarding the safety of laparoscopic surgery in patients who have colon cancer are valid for laparoscopic rectal cancer. Although there have been several clinical trials testing the equivalence of laparoscopic colectomy in the setting of curable colon cancer, few studies are available to examine the same question in rectal cancer. What is relevant in rectal cancer is whether laparoscopic techniques can achieve tumor-free margins with the same rate as open surgery.[32] Pelvic dissection might be facilitated by laparoscopic equipment, and access to the deep pelvis with lighting and visualization might be superior to open surgery in some cases. This has not been proven in diverse practice settings. An additional concern is the ability to achieve distal stapling because of the limits of current instrumentation. These issues are being addressed by a prospective, randomized trial conducted by the American College of Surgeons Oncology Group (ACOSOG).[33] The ACOSOG Z6051 trial is a multicenter, phase III, randomized, clinical trial with the primary objective of showing that laparoscopic-assisted resection for rectal cancer is not inferior to open rectal resection, based on the composite primary end point of oncologic factors that indicate a safe and feasible operation. The end point of this noninferiority trial is based on detailed and standardized pathologic evaluation of the specimen, including circumferential and distal margins and the completeness of the total mesorectal excision. The primary end point is a novel, surrogate end point for long-term oncologic outcome that reduces both the necessary accrual target of the trial and its time to maturation. The secondary end points include patient-related benefits (blood loss, length of stay, pain medicine use), 2-year local recurrence, and QOL. This noninferiority trial is projected to enroll 650 eligible patients in the United States and Canada. The trial is sponsored by the NCI. Further details and contact information can be obtained from the following Web site: http://www.cancer.gov/clinicaltrials/ACOSOG-Z605.

Available data allow a summary of the main points that should be considered to pursue a correct management of patients who have colon cancer, when they are considered suitable for a laparoscopic operation:

1. Accurate preoperative defining of the extent of the disease is a prerequisite.
2. Preoperative tattooing of the lesion with colonoscopy aids in the localization of the tumor during the procedure.
3. Dense adhesions or extensive disease that prevents accurate identification of the vital structures and increase the risk of complications should cause the surgeon to convert early to an open procedure.
4. Placement of a ureteral stent or conversion to open surgery should be considered when there is difficulty in locating 1 or both ureters as a result of inflammation or tumor in the retroperitoneum.
5. It is essential to perform a complete oncological resection. This procedure includes adequate mobilization, high vascular ligation, satisfactory lymph node harvest, and negative resection margins. Intracorporeal ligation is sometimes required to achieve high vascular ligation.

6. Conversion (conversion rates and reasons for conversion from trials are shown in **Table 7**). In general, the initial exploration should determine the feasibility of laparoscopic resection to assess early whether conversion is indicated and then to convert promptly to save time, frustration, and prevent possible complications; early conversion indications should include[26]: massive adhesions, small bowel fixed in pelvis, bulky disease, unusual anatomy, and unexpected findings.

FUTURE PROSPECTS: ROBOTICS AND NATURAL-ORIFICE TRANSLUMINAL ENDOSCOPIC SURGERY

Laparoscopic surgery has reached a comfortable plateau. Practitioners are catching up with the technology. Laparoscopic techniques and tools have penetrated the practice in many surgical arenas, and virtually all trainees now have exposure and experience in minimally invasive surgery. The comfort zone has widened and incremental progress is occurring everywhere. Soon it will be time for the introduction of robotic and natural-orifice surgery.

Successful telerobotic-assisted laparoscopic sigmoid and right colectomies were first reported by Weber and colleagues[34] in 2002, in which dissection and mobilization were performed with robotic assistance. D'Annibale and colleagues[35] reported the results of 53 robotic colorectal surgeries in 2004 and concluded that the outcomes were similar to those of laparoscopic surgery. Short-term outcomes of a randomized pilot study by Baik and colleagues[36] comparing robotic-assisted low anterior resection with laparoscopic low anterior resection confirmed the safety and feasibility of robotics in colorectal surgery. Robotic-assisted surgery (Da Vinci robot) offers many advantages compared with laparoscopic surgery, including three-dimensional visualization, increased degrees of freedom of movement, absence of fulcrum effect, reduced fatigue, and elimination of tremor, plus improved ergonomics for the surgeon.[35] The biggest drawback for robotics is the high cost. Current drawbacks for robotics include the absence of tactile sensation, the lengthy time required for set up, and the initial cost of the equipment. Given the absence of compelling gains, the robot has not become popular in practice.

The natural-orifice specimen extraction technique has been performed in colon and rectal surgery specimen extraction through transanal and transvaginal routes in the

Table 7 Conversion rate and reasons for conversion from LAC to OC				
	COST	COLOR	CLASSIC	Barcelona
Conversion rate (%)	21	17	29	11
Reasons for Conversion (%)				
Advanced disease	25	42.8	—	—
Complicated disease	3	—	—	—
Inadequate margin of resection	4	—	21	—
No visualization of critical structure	13	5.4	—	—
Unable to mobilize colon	11	—	61	—
Adhesion	15	10.9	—	—
Intraoperative complication	4	8.7	—	—
Obesity	—	—	8	—
Other	24	31.8	—	—

recent past, and was considered a prequel to natural-orifice transluminal endoscopic surgery (NOTES).[37] NOTES is a concept that is gaining enthusiasm. NOTES approaches the internal viscera through natural openings such as the mouth (stomach), the anus, and the vagina. NOTES was first performed in India by Reddy and Rao in a burned patient for whom abdominal incision was not feasible.[38] Initial studies were performed mainly on animal models.[39] The Natural Orifice Surgery Consortium for Assessment for Research (NOSCAR) was formed in 2005 and identified the potential barriers to the clinical practice of NOTES and set guidelines for future research and development.[40] Patients prefer to undergo NOTES rather than laparoscopic cholecystectomy because of a lack of pain (99%) and external scarring (89%).[41] The potential advantages of NOTES are no scars, less pain, fewer wound complications, earlier mobility and recovery,[39] and the potential to offer therapy outside the operating room.[42]

It might be argued that natural-orifice surgery is the logical extension of the current laparoscopic approach, especially considering that the target organ, the bowel, and the natural orifice, the anus, are continuous structures. Although the realization of natural-orifice surgery is not expected for several years, particularly for colon cancer treatment, this reality is substantially closer because of the lessons learned from laparoscopic cancer trials. Thousands of patients agreed to participate in colon cancer trials, with unknown oncologic results, and this has provided a great deal of information about the importance of postoperative pain and discomfort, scars, QOL, and duration of recovery in patient decision making.

SUMMARY

As a result of several years of trials and investigations, laparoscopic colectomy for colon cancer is now considered an acceptable and safe alternative to traditional open techniques. Four large randomized trials (Barcelona, COST, COLOR, CLASSIC) have shown the noninferiority of laparoscopic colectomy in overall survival, DFS, and overall and local recurrences. Laparoscopic surgery is associated with better short-term outcomes such as shorter hospital stay, shorter duration of ileus, less narcotic usefulness and postoperative pain, and a faster postoperative recovery. The procedures are also safe and feasible in elderly patients. Hand-assisted laparoscopic colectomy is a recent hybrid technique that could reduce learning time, and its role has been established in more challenging procedures. Future prospects include robotic and natural-orifice surgery.

REFERENCES

1. Lacy AM, García-Valdecasas JC, Delgado S, et al. Laparoscopy-assisted colectomy versus open colectomy for treatment of non-metastatic colon cancer: a randomised trial. Lancet 2002;359(9325):2224-9.
2. Lacy AM, Delgado S, Castells A, et al. The long-term results of a randomized clinical trial of laparoscopy-assisted versus open surgery for colon cancer. Ann Surg 2008;248(1):1-7.
3. Nelson H, COST Study Group. A comparison of laparoscopically assisted and open colectomy for colon cancer. N Engl J Med 2004;350(20):2050-9.
4. Fleshman J, Sargent DJ, Green E, et al. Laparoscopic colectomy for cancer is not inferior to open surgery based on 5-year data from the COST Study Group trial. Ann Surg 2007;246(4):655-62.

5. Veldkamp R, Kuhry E, Hop WC, et al. Laparoscopic surgery versus open surgery for colon cancer: short-term outcomes of a randomised trial. Lancet Oncol 2005; 6:477–84.

6. Buunen M, Veldkamp R, Hop WC, et al. Survival after laparoscopic surgery versus open surgery for colon cancer: long-term outcome of a randomised clinical trial. Lancet Oncol 2009;10(1):44–52.

7. Guillou PJ, Quirke P, Thorpe H, et al. Short-term endpoints of conventional versus laparoscopic-assisted surgery in patients with colorectal cancer (MRC CLASICC trial): multicentre, randomised controlled trial. Lancet 2005;365:1718–26.

8. Jayne DG, Guillou PJ, Thorpe H, et al. Randomized trial of laparoscopic-assisted resection of colorectal carcinoma: 3-year results of the UK MRC CLASICC Trial Group. J Clin Oncol 2007;25(21):3061–8.

9. Liang JT, Huang KC, Lai HS, et al. Oncologic results of laparoscopic versus conventional open surgery for stage II or III left-sided colon cancers: a randomized controlled trial. Ann Surg Oncol 2007;14(1):109–17.

10. Tjandra JJ, Chan MK. Systematic review on the short-term outcome of laparoscopic resection for colon and rectosigmoid cancer. Colorectal Dis 2006;8(5): 375–88.

11. Schwenk W, Haase O, Neudecker J, et al. Short term benefits for laparoscopic colorectal resection. Cochrane Database Syst Rev 2005;3:CD003145.

12. Bilimoria KY, Bentrem DJ, Merkow RP, et al. Laparoscopic-assisted vs. open colectomy for cancer: comparison of short-term outcomes from 121 hospitals. J Gastrointest Surg 2008;12(11):2001–9.

13. Weeks JC, Nelson H, Gelber S, et al. Short-term quality-of-life outcomes following laparoscopic-assisted colectomy vs open colectomy for colon cancer: a randomized trial. JAMA 2002;287(3):321–8.

14. Sackett DL. Rules of evidence and clinical recommendations on the use of antithrombotic agents. Chest 1989;95(Suppl 2):2S–4S.

15. Frazee RC, Roberts JW, Okeson GC, et al. Open versus laparoscopic cholecystectomy. A comparison of postoperative pulmonary function. Ann Surg 1991; 213(6):651–3.

16. Stocchi L, Nelson H, Young-Fadok TM, et al. Safety and advantages of laparoscopic vs. open colectomy in the elderly: matched-control study. Dis Colon Rectum 2000;43(3):326–32.

17. Wise WE Jr, Padmanabhan A, Meesig DM, et al. Abdominal colon and rectal operations in the elderly. Dis Colon Rectum 1991;34(11):959–63.

18. Jacobs M, Verdeja JC, Goldstein HS. Minimally invasive colon resection (laparoscopic colectomy). Surg Laparosc Endosc 1991;1(3):144–50.

19. Johnstone PA, Rohde DC, Swartz SE, et al. Port site recurrences after laparoscopic and thoracoscopic procedures in malignancy. J Clin Oncol 1996;14(6): 1950–6.

20. Restrepo JI, Stocchi L, Nelson H, et al. Laparoscopic ultrasonography: a training model. Dis Colon Rectum 2001;44(5):632–7.

21. Marchesa P, Milsom JW, Hale JC, et al. Intraoperative laparoscopic liver ultrasonography for staging of colorectal cancer. Initial experience. Dis Colon Rectum 1996;39(Suppl 10):S73–8.

22. Bonjer HJ, Hop WC, Nelson H, et al. Laparoscopically assisted vs open colectomy for colon cancer: a meta-analysis. Arch Surg 2007;142(3):298–303.

23. Bernstein MA, Dawson JW, Reissman P, et al. Is complete laparoscopic colectomy superior to laparoscopic assisted colectomy? Am Surg 1996;62(6):507–11.

24. Liang JT, Lai HS, Huang KC, et al. Comparison of medial-to-lateral versus traditional lateral-to-medial laparoscopic dissection sequences for resection of rectosigmoid cancers: randomized controlled clinical trial. World J Surg 2003;27(2): 190–6.
25. Rotholtz NA, Bun ME, Tessio M, et al. Laparoscopic colectomy: medial versus lateral approach. Surg Laparosc Endosc Percutan Tech 2009;19(1):43–7.
26. Young-Fadok TM, Nelson H. Laparoscopic right colectomy: five-step procedure. Dis Colon Rectum 2000;43(2):267–71.
27. Steele SR, Brown TA, Rush RM, et al. Laparoscopic vs open colectomy for colon cancer: results from a large nationwide population-based analysis. J Gastrointest Surg 2008;12(3):583–91.
28. Kemp JA, Finlayson SR. Nationwide trends in laparoscopic colectomy from 2000 to 2004. Surg Endosc 2008;22(5):1181–7.
29. Cima RR, Pattana-arun J, Larson DW, et al. Experience with 969 minimal access colectomies: the role of hand-assisted laparoscopy in expanding minimally invasive surgery for complex colectomies. J Am Coll Surg 2008;206(5): 946–50.
30. Ozturk E, Kiran RP, Geisler DP, et al. Hand-assisted laparoscopic colectomy: benefits of laparoscopic colectomy at no extra cost. J Am Coll Surg 2009; 209(2):242–7.
31. Marcello PW, Fleshman JW, Milsom JW, et al. Hand-assisted laparoscopic vs. laparoscopic colorectal surgery: a multicenter, prospective, randomized trial. Dis Colon Rectum 2008;51(6):818–26.
32. Boller AM, Nelson H. Colon and rectal cancer: laparoscopic or open? Clin Cancer Res 2007;13(22 Pt 2):6894s–6s.
33. Soop M, Nelson H. Laparoscopic-assisted proctectomy for rectal cancer: on trial. Ann Surg Oncol 2008;15(9):2357–9.
34. Weber PA, Merola S, Wasielewski A, et al. Telerobotic-assisted laparoscopic right and sigmoid colectomies for benign disease. Dis Colon Rectum 2002;45(12): 1689–94 [discussion: 1695–6].
35. D'Annibale A, Morpurgo E, Fiscon V, et al. Robotic and laparoscopic surgery for treatment of colorectal diseases. Dis Colon Rectum 2004;47(12):2162–8.
36. Baik SH, Ko YT, Kang CM, et al. Robotic tumor-specific mesorectal excision of rectal cancer: short-term outcome of a pilot randomized trial. Surg Endosc 2008;22(7):1601–8.
37. Palanivelu C, Rangarajan M, Jategaonkar PA, et al. An innovative technique for colorectal specimen retrieval: a new era of "natural orifice specimen extraction" (N.O.S.E). Dis Colon Rectum 2008;51(7):1120–4.
38. Baron TH. Natural orifice transluminal endoscopic surgery. Br J Surg 2007;94(1): 1–2.
39. Al-Akash M, Boyle E, Tanner WA. NOTES: the progression of a novel and emerging technique. Surg Oncol 2009;18(2):95–103.
40. Rattner D, Kalloo A. ASGE/SAGES working group on natural orifice translumenal endoscopic surgery. October 2005. Surg Endosc 2006;20(2):329–33.
41. Varadarajulu S, Tamhane A, Drelichman ER. Patient perception of natural orifice transluminal endoscopic surgery as a technique for cholecystectomy. Gastrointest Endosc 2008;67(6):854–60.
42. Onders RP, McGee MF, Marks J, et al. Natural orifice transluminal endoscopic surgery (NOTES) as a diagnostic tool in the intensive care unit. Surg Endosc 2007;21(4):681–3.

Laparoscopy for Rectal Cancer

Govind Nandakumar, MD[a,b],*, James W. Fleshman, MD[b]

KEYWORDS

• Laparoscopy • Rectal cancer • Total mesorectal excision
• Colon cancer

Following the success and wide implementation of laparoscopic cholecystectomy, reports on the use of laparoscopy for colon resections soon appeared.[1] Unfortunately, due to initial concerns regarding the oncologic quality of the operation and reports of port site implants, there was hesitance in the application of laparoscopy to colon and rectal cancer. Between 1994 and 2004 there were multiple randomized control trials conducted to study the use of laparoscopy for the treatment of colon cancer.[2] The data on colon cancer have since matured, suggesting that laparoscopy offers short-term benefits with no compromise on the oncologic outcome. On the other hand, the number of large multicenter randomized trials on the use of laparoscopy for rectal cancer is limited.[3–6] The dearth of quality data is probably secondary to the technical challenges of working within the confines of the bony pelvis while adhering to the principles of total mesorectal excision (TME), autonomic nerve preservation, and maintenance of adequate circumferential and distal margin. This review provides an update on the current and upcoming data on the use of laparoscopy for the treatment of rectal cancer. The authors also briefly review the critical areas of technique that affect oncologic resection and the data on the use of robotics for rectal cancer.

LAPAROSCOPIC COLON CANCER SURGERY

Laparoscopy is now an established technique for the treatment of colon cancer at major centers. Mature data from the COST, COLOR, ALCCaS, and CLASICC trials have clarified that the oncologic outcome and 3- to 5-year survival can be maintained while providing significant short-term benefits.[3,7–9] Today, with compelling evidence from the large multicenter trials, there is increasing use of laparoscopy for the

The authors received no financial support for this work.
The authors have nothing to disclose.
[a] Department of Surgery, Weill Cornell Medical College, 525 East 68th Street, Box 172, New York, NY 10065, USA
[b] Section of Colon and Rectal Surgery, Washington University School of Medicine, 660 South Euclid Avenue, Box 8109, St Louis, MO 63110, USA
* Corresponding author. Department of Surgery, Weill Cornell Medical College, 525 East 68th Street, Box 172, New York, NY 10065.
E-mail address: doctorgovind@gmail.com

treatment of colon cancer, and with standardized techniques laparoscopic colon cancer surgery is being used by surgeons in the community as well.[10,11]

LAPAROSCOPY FOR RECTAL CANCER

In stark contrast to the robust data for colon cancer that have developed over the last decade, there are limited quality data on the use of laparoscopy for the treatment of rectal cancer. The United Kingdom Medical Research Council (UK MRC) CLASICC trial is the only major colon cancer trial that did not exclude rectal cancer patients. In the CLASICC trial, a randomized trial involving 27 centers in the United Kingdom, 242 rectal dissections (randomized 2:1, laparoscopic to open) were performed by surgeons who had completed a minimum of 20 laparoscopic colon resections. Even this specialized group of surgeons had a 34% conversion rate to open operation for completion of rectal dissection. Tumor fixation and uncertainty of margins were the 2 most common reasons for conversion.[3] The CLASICC trial offers the highest level of evidence for the use of laparoscopy to treat rectal cancer.[3,12] In addition, randomized controlled single-institution trials have shown favorable outcomes for short-term results and oncologic parameters.[5,13–15] The data from large single-center trials and case series are reviewed in 2 meta-analyses[16,17] and Cochrane reviews of the data.[18,19]

TECHNIQUE

The authors' preoperative preparation of the patient includes a mechanical bowel preparation, betadine rectal wash in the operating room, preoperative antibiotics, and deep venous thrombosis prophylaxis with perioperative low molecular weight heparin. The patient is placed in a modified lithotomy position on a cocooning bean bag secured to the operating table with Velcro or safety straps, and padded to prevent pressure injury. It is critical to ensure that the thighs are in line with the torso to avoid interference with the laparoscopic instruments. Pneumoperitoneum is achieved using a Veress needle or an open technique. If a hand-assist device is used, an 8-cm lower midline or pfannenstiel incision is used to gain access.

One 10-mm trocar is placed at the umbilicus for the camera. After achieving pneumoperitoneum, a second 10-mm suprapubic trocar is placed, which is useful for retraction and passage of the Endo-Cutter stapling device. Two 5-mm trocars are placed under direct vision along the right anterior axillary line, the first 2 finger breadths inferior to the costal margin and the second 2 finger breadths superior to the right anterior superior iliac spine. One 5-mm trocar is placed as lateral as possible in the left anterior axillary line.

The patient is placed in Trendelenburg position and tilted to have the left side up. A 10-mm laparoscopic grasper is used to identify and expose the inferior mesenteric artery (IMA), which is the only artery arising from the aorta above the sacral promontory and below the duodenum. Care is taken to retract the small bowel medially so that the entire sigmoid mesentery is in clear view. With upward traction on the IMA, the peritoneum is incised along the inferior border of the vessel. The retroperitoneal window is developed medial to lateral, and the left ureter is clearly identified. The inferior mesenteric vein is identified in a similar fashion between the duodenum and the IMA, running parallel to the aorta at the base of the left colon mesentery. Mesenteric fat is dissected off the vessels to skeletonize the artery and vein completely. The vessels are divided with either an energy source or a stapling device. The authors' preference is to use to the 5-mm ENSEAL device, applying 3 overlapping burns on the vessel and dividing in the middle. Prior to division, it is essential to ensure that the ureter is not adherent to the posterior surface of the mesentery along its entire course and that the hypogastric nerves are free of the IMA. The sigmoid colon is then freed off its lateral attachments and dissection is carried along the splenic flexure. The retroperitoneum is seen as a purple layer adherent to the mesentery posteriorly. With appropriate traction and countertraction, the left colon mesentery is dissected off the retroperitoneum up to the tail of the pancreas. The patient is placed in reverse Trendelenburg, head-up, position. The avascular plane along the inferior border of the pancreas, just anterior to the pancreas, is incised to gain entry into the lesser sac. The splenic flexure is mobilized completely to gain as much mobility of the colon as possible.

The patient is returned to Trendelenburg position, placed in a neutral right/left position, and attention is then turned to the pelvis. The rectum is retracted anteriorly and out of the pelvis to expose the avascular plane posterior to the mesorectum. The hook cautery is used to develop the posterior plane as far distally as possible and laterally along the pelvic side walls in a semicircular midline motion that follows the curve of the pelvis. The right and left hypogastric nerves are identified and protected. With constant traction on the rectum opposite to the side of dissection, the lateral peritoneal attachments are released. The anterolateral ligaments are then divided with the hook cautery using the areolar tissue plane as the guide for dissection. The mesorectum is dissected to at least 5 cm below the distal level of the tumor.

If the patient is to have a low anterior resection, an endoscopic stapler is placed in the suprapubic port. The mesorectum is divided at right angles to the rectum at the appropriate level using the energy device to facilitate transection of the rectum. An endoscopic gastrointestinal stapler is used to divide the rectum at the desired level 5 cm below the tumor. A stapler that articulates is useful, and often requires 2 or more applications to transect the rectum. There is evidence that minimizing the number of stapler fires for rectal transection may decrease the incidence of anastomotic leaks.[20] The specimen is exteriorized through the ileostomy site or a separate incision. The colon is divided in the standard fashion and the anvil of the circular stapling device placed in the proximal colon. The shaft of the end-to-end anastomosis (EEA) stapler is then placed in the rectum and the anastomosis completed under direct visualization.

If the patient is scheduled to have an abdominoperineal resection, the laparoscopic dissection is carried as far distally as possible. The proximal colon is divided and the specimen left in the pelvis. The trocar sites are closed, and the colostomy placed through the left lower quadrant and matured. The patient is then placed in a prone jack-knife position for the perineal dissection, specimen extraction, and closure.

The specimen is evaluated both macroscopically and microscopically by a specialized pathologist to grade the quality of resection. The specimen is examined by the surgeon and pathologist and inked in the operating room. Quirke and colleagues[21,22] outlined a protocol to systematically evaluate the macroscopic quality of the TME specimen. The completeness of the mesorectal envelope after the dissection has been shown to correlate with local recurrence and cancer outcomes by the Dutch TME studies.[23,24] A new classification system of the mesorectal planes was recently described: MA-0 (complete), MA-1 (incomplete but mostly intact), and MA-2 (violated, inadequate mesorectal excision).[25] The distal and circumferential margins should be assessed by an expert pathologist.[26] The importance of the circumferential resection margin has been highlighted by Quirke and colleagues over the years,[23,24,27] and documentation of circumferential resection margin involvement is an independent prognostic factor for rectal cancer.[28,29]

SHORT-TERM OUTCOMES

The mean operating time for laparoscopic resection of rectal cancer has been reported to be between 180 and 220 minutes, with most large series reporting longer operative times for the laparoscopic techniques.[30] There are few reports of equivalent or shorter operative times for laparoscopic rectal resection.[13,31] Most comparative studies and randomized trials report lower blood loss in the laparoscopic group.[30] A recent Cochrane review of the literature confirmed that laparoscopic proctectomy is associated with a lower blood loss.[18] In the CLASICC trial, there was a decrease in median length of stay from 13 to 11 days with no significant difference in the time to first bowel movement and resumption of normal oral diet. Neither the meta-analyses nor the CLASICC trial reported any difference in 30-day mortality. The 2 meta-analyses showed more convincing short-term advantages including a lower incidence of wound infection (0% vs 14%),[16] overall morbidity (21% vs 28%),[17] return of stoma function (1.5 days earlier), and length of hospital stay (2.7 days shorter) for the laparoscopic group.[16] A Cochrane review of 80 studies that included 4224 patients found that laparoscopic TME was associated with quicker return to normal diet, less pain, less narcotic use, and less immune response. The Cochrane review reported a trend toward longer operative time and higher operative cost.[18]

ONCOLOGIC OUTCOMES

TME has decreased the incidence of recurrence after proctectomy for rectal cancer.[32,33] Adherence to the principles of TME with laparoscopic surgery seems critical in maintaining a good oncologic outcome. The best available markers for a successful TME remain evaluation of the quality of the TME specimen, uninvolved circumferential resection margin (CRM), uninvolved distal margin, and maximal lymph node harvest. Even though the 2006 meta-analysis showed no difference in overall oncologic outcomes between laparoscopic and open approaches, the investigators recommended multicenter randomized trials.[16] The rates of positive CRM were lower overall and were not different between the laparoscopic and open groups.[16]

One concerning trend noted in the CLASICC trial was a numerically larger, though statistically insignificant, rate of positive CRM in laparoscopic-assisted anterior resection compared with open resection (12% vs 6%).[3] However, the higher CRM positivity in the anterior resection arm did not translate into a higher local recurrence rate at the 3-year follow up.[12] The overall 3-year survival rate was 68%, with no difference in the survival rate or quality of life between the laparoscopic and open arms. On subset analysis, there was no difference in overall survival between the 2 modalities among patients who underwent an abdominoperineal resection or anterior resection. Of note, the rate of complete TME was higher in the laparoscopic group than in the open group, supporting the argument that laparoscopy may offer better visualization and magnification in the pelvis.

A study specifically designed to assess the macroscopic quality of rectal resections randomized 72 patients to laparoscopic versus open proctectomy. Laparoscopic proctectomy was associated with a lower anastomosis ($P<.001$) and a higher likelihood of having an intact visceral fascia.[34] Two randomized controlled trials and other large nonrandomized comparative trials found no difference in the number of lymph nodes retrieved between the laparoscopic and open rectal resections.[6,14,35–38]

BLADDER AND SEXUAL FUNCTION

Preservation of pelvic nerves during TME is important to maintain bladder and sexual function. Despite efforts to identify and preserve pelvic nerves during TME, the incidence of bladder and sexual dysfunction has been reported to range between 0% to 12% and 10% to 35%, respectively.[39–41] Although a beneficial relationship has not been established as yet, the magnification offered with laparoscopic dissection may facilitate the identification of pelvic nerves.[42,43] In the CLASICC trial, bladder and sexual function were not found to be statistically different between laparoscopic and open TME. Overall 65% of patients were able to void without difficulty. Male sexual function and erectile function tended to be worse in the laparoscopic group than in the open group, though not statistically significant ($P = .063$). The investigators attributed the difference to the higher number of TME dissections in the laparoscopic group (80% in the laparoscopic group vs 63% in the open group).[40] On multivariate analysis of the CLASICC data, TME and conversion to open surgery were both independent predictors of postoperative male sexual dysfunction.[40] A recent retrospective review of laparoscopic proctectomy reported a bladder and sexual dysfunction rate of 6%. The investigators attributed their superior results to the experience of their surgeons and highlighted the steep "learning curve" for laparoscopic proctectomy.[44] Preservation of pelvic nerves is clearly an important aspect of proctectomy, and upcoming studies will clarify whether laparoscopy can offer improved identification and preservation of pelvic nerves.

CURRENT AND UPCOMING TRIALS

There are several large multicenter randomized prospective studies under way to evaluate the role of laparoscopy in the treatment of rectal cancer. The European Colon Cancer Laparoscopic or Open Resection (COLOR) II trial is a multicenter randomized control trial comparing outcomes of laparoscopic and open resections for rectal carcinoma with a curative intent. The COLOR II trial started accruing in June 2003, and involves 27 centers across Europe, Canada, and South Korea with a primary outcome measure of 3-year locoregional recurrence. While some preliminary feasibility data are available from this study, interim analysis of rectal cancer patients is ongoing and should be reported soon.[45] The Japan Clinical Oncology Group (JCOG) study 0404 started accruing patients with T3 and T4 tumors in 2004, and includes tumors in the rectosigmoid.[46] In the United States, the American College of Surgeons Oncology Group trial (ACOSOG) Z6051 is under way and should provide good-quality data on the oncologic outcome of laparoscopy for rectal cancer. The study began in August 2008 with a goal of enrolling 480 patients comparing open (includes hybrid laparoscopic assisted) versus laparoscopic (includes robotic) resection for rectal cancer. Primary end points include CRM, distal margin, and completeness of the TME. Secondary end points include overall and disease-free survival and local recurrence at 2 years, quality of life, sexual function, bladder function, and stoma function.[47] The UK MRC CLASICC trial should have 5-year oncologic and survival data shortly.[3,12] Other registered international trials include one in Korea and one in Singapore.[48,49]

In the absence of 5-year survival data, laparoscopic proctectomy should be offered only in the setting of a trial. To collect data in a systematic fashion, the American Society of Colon and Rectal Surgeons (ASCRS) and the Society of Gastrointestinal and Endoscopic Surgeons (SAGES) issued a joint statement encouraging surgeons to perform laparoscopic proctectomy for cancer in the setting of a trial.[50]

HAND-ASSISTED LAPAROSCOPY

The use of a hand-assist device during laparoscopic colon and rectal surgery mitigates some of the technical challenges of the procedure. Proponents of the hand-assist approach argue that because an extraction site is required for specimen removal, this incision can be used to facilitate dissection. Data from a multicenter randomized control trial showed shorter operative times, while maintaining the short-term benefits of laparoscopy for left, total abdominal, and total proctocolectomies.[51]A single-center randomized control trial found no difference in the short-term outcome between straight laparoscopic and hand-assisted colectomy for cancer.[4] A systematic review and meta-analysis that included colectomy performed for benign and malignant disease found no difference in the short-term outcome between laparoscopic and hand-assisted surgery.[52] Hand-assisted laparoscopy is an important minimally invasive tool that aids in training new surgeons, expands the use of laparoscopy to technically challenging cases that might have previously been approached without laparoscopy, and expedites the operation in the daily list of a busy surgeon. A randomized control trial is under way to specifically evaluate "pure laparoscopic" versus hand-assisted laparoscopic proctectomy for rectal cancer.[53]

ROBOTIC PROCTECTOMY

Operating within the confines of the pelvis to perform a good TME for cancer is technically demanding with the laparoscope. Robotic systems are useful when the operative field is small and a precise dissection is required to successfully complete the operation. There have been recent reports looking at the feasibility of robotic proctectomy for rectal cancer. The potential advantage derives from the direct entry angle of the robotic instruments into the pelvis, which gives the surgeon the view and angle of dissection as if sitting on the patient's chest. Initial case series have reported short-term outcomes similar to laparoscopic proctectomy.[54–56] Baik and colleagues[54] reported on 56 patients who underwent robotic proctectomy for rectal cancer. The conversion rate to open was 0% in the robotic group compared with 10% in the laparoscopic group, with a higher number of "complete TME" in the robotic group. However, these trends were not statistically significant. Robotic proctectomy may offer improved visualization of the pelvic nerves and decrease the rate of bladder and sexual dysfunction. It is noteworthy that laparoscopic surgeons who work in the pelvis commonly have lower back problems, and robotic systems might create a more ergonomically friendly environment for the surgeon during proctectomy.[57] However, robotic proctectomy is a new technique under development that requires more rigorous studies before its use can be accepted as standard therapy for the treatment of rectal cancer. Robotic and laparoscopic procedures are being included in the laparoscopic arm of the ACOSOG Z6051 trial, and other trials comparing laparoscopy and robotic techniques are in the planning stages.

TRAINING AND CREDENTIALING

Early literature reported the learning curve for laparoscopic colon surgery to be 20 to 50 cases.[58–60] The COST and CLASICC trials required a minimum of 20 cases and a validated video for surgeons to be credentialed to perform laparoscopic colon surgery.[3,4] Extrapolating from the COST and CLASICC experience, the ASCRS and SAGES recommended 20 as the minimum number of laparoscopic colon resections to be credentialed for colon cancer resections.[61]

Laparoscopic rectal cancer surgery is more technically demanding than laparoscopic colon surgery. Park and colleagues[62] retrospectively performed a multidimensional analysis of the learning curve for laparoscopic rectal cancer from December 2002 to December 2007. The series of a single surgeon was divided into 4 periods based on the number of operations. The conversion rate decreased from 5.6% in the first period to 1.5% in the fourth period. Anastomotic leak rates decreased from 10.3% in the first period to 1.6% in the fourth period. A similar trend was seen in the local recurrence rate (22.9% in the first period to 4.4% in the fourth period for stage

I–III cancers). These data need to be interpreted with certain caveats—the selection bias in these groups is unclear and fewer patients in the first group received radiation. Nevertheless, the investigators concluded that the learning curve for laparoscopic rectal cancer surgery changed significantly with surgeon experience. This study also hypothesized that the oncologic learning curve may be steeper than the technical learning curve for laparoscopic rectal cancer surgery. In the MRC CLASICC trial, conversion was higher in the rectal cancer cohort and decreased from 38% in year 1 to 16% in year 6.[12] The decrease in the conversion rate was likely related to improved surgeon experience and patient selection.

Although 20 cases might serve as a minimum learning curve, it is difficult to recommend an absolute number. Participation in courses sponsored by organizations such as the ASCRS facilitates adoption of laparoscopic techniques in clinical practice.[63] Credentialing for laparoscopic proctectomy, robotic proctectomy, and NOTES (natural orifice trans-endoluminal surgery) will remain a challenge as these techniques develop. Video credentialing, random video audit, and standardized pathologic grading of the TME specimens can assure quality of technique.

SUMMARY

Laparoscopic rectal cancer surgery is technically challenging, but feasible for surgeons who have experience with open rectal cancer surgery and advanced laparoscopy. Data from several large international multicenter trials that are currently under way will be needed to clarify the oncologic and long-term safety of laparoscopic proctectomy for rectal cancer. As we continue to define the role of laparoscopy in the treatment of rectal cancer, laparoscopic resections should be performed in the setting of well-constructed trials. Robotic and endoluminal techniques are under investigation, and will likely be essential tools for future minimally invasive colorectal surgeons. Training, credentialing, and quality control are important as we apply these new technologies to the treatment of rectal cancer.

REFERENCES

1. Jacobs M, Verdeja JC, Goldstein HS. Minimally invasive colon resection (laparoscopic colectomy). Surg Laparosc Endosc 1991;1(3):144–50.
2. Soop M, Nelson H. Is laparoscopic resection appropriate for colorectal adenocarcinoma? Adv Surg 2008;42:205–17.
3. Guillou PJ, Quirke P, Thorpe H, et al. Short-term endpoints of conventional versus laparoscopic-assisted surgery in patients with colorectal cancer (MRC CLASICC trial): multicentre, randomised controlled trial. Lancet 2005;365(9472):1718–26.
4. Laparoscopically assisted colectomy is as safe and effective as open colectomy in people with colon cancer Abstracted from: Nelson H, Sargent D, Wieand HS, et al; for the Clinical Outcomes of Surgical Therapy Study Group. A comparison of laparoscopically assisted and open colectomy for colon cancer. N Engl J Med 2004;350:2050–9. Cancer Treat Rev 2004;30(8):707–9.
5. Leung KL, Kwok SP, Lam SC, et al. Laparoscopic resection of rectosigmoid carcinoma: prospective randomised trial. Lancet 2004;363(9416):1187–92.
6. Ng SS, Leung KL, Lee JF, et al. Laparoscopic-assisted versus open abdominoperineal resection for low rectal cancer: a prospective randomized trial. Ann Surg Oncol 2008;15(9):2418–25.
7. Fleshman J, Sargent DJ, Green E, et al. Laparoscopic colectomy for cancer is not inferior to open surgery based on 5-year data from the COST Study Group trial. Ann Surg 2007;246(4):655–62 [discussion: 662–4].

8. Buunen M, Veldkamp R, Hop WC, et al. Survival after laparoscopic surgery versus open surgery for colon cancer: long-term outcome of a randomised clinical trial. Lancet Oncol 2009;10(1):44–52.
9. Hewett PJ, Allardyce RA, Bagshaw PF, et al. Short-term outcomes of the Australasian randomized clinical study comparing laparoscopic and conventional open surgical treatments for colon cancer: the ALCCaS trial. Ann Surg 2008;248(5):728–38.
10. Scala A, Huang A, Dowson HM, et al. Laparoscopic colorectal surgery—results from 200 patients. Colorectal Dis 2007;9(8):701–5.
11. Fiscon V, Frigo F, Migliorini G, et al. Laparoscopic colon resection by a single general surgeon in a community hospital: a review of 200 consecutive cases. J Laparoendosc Adv Surg Tech A 2009;19(1):13–7.
12. Jayne DG, Guillou PJ, Thorpe H, et al. Randomized trial of laparoscopic-assisted resection of colorectal carcinoma: 3-year results of the UK MRC CLASICC Trial Group. J Clin Oncol 2007;25(21):3061–8.
13. Araujo SE, da Silva eSousa AH Jr, de Campos FG, et al. Conventional approach × laparoscopic abdominoperineal resection for rectal cancer treatment after neoadjuvant chemoradiation: results of a prospective randomized trial. Rev Hosp Clin Fac Med Sao Paulo 2003;58(3):133–40.
14. Braga M, Frasson M, Vignali A, et al. Laparoscopic resection in rectal cancer patients: outcome and cost-benefit analysis. Dis Colon Rectum 2007;50(4):464–71.
15. Feliciotti F, Guerrieri M, Paganini AM, et al. Long-term results of laparoscopic versus open resections for rectal cancer for 124 unselected patients. Surg Endosc 2003;17(10):1530–5.
16. Aziz O, Constantinides V, Tekkis PP, et al. Laparoscopic versus open surgery for rectal cancer: a meta-analysis. Ann Surg Oncol 2006;13(3):413–24.
17. Gao F, Cao YF, Chen LS. Meta-analysis of short-term outcomes after laparoscopic resection for rectal cancer. Int J Colorectal Dis 2006;21(7):652–6.
18. Breukink S, Pierie J, Wiggers T. Laparoscopic versus open total mesorectal excision for rectal cancer. Cochrane Database Syst Rev 2006;4:CD005200.
19. Kuhry E, Schwenk W, Gaupset R, et al. Long-term outcome of laparoscopic surgery for colorectal cancer: a Cochrane systematic review of randomised controlled trials. Cancer Treat Rev 2008;34(6):498–504.
20. Kim JS, Cho SY, Min BS, et al. Risk factors for anastomotic leakage after laparoscopic intracorporeal colorectal anastomosis with a double stapling technique. J Am Coll Surg 2009;209(6):694–701.
21. Quirke P, Durdey P, Dixon MF, et al. Local recurrence of rectal adenocarcinoma due to inadequate surgical resection. Histopathological study of lateral tumour spread and surgical excision. Lancet 1986;2(8514):996–9.
22. Quirke P, Dixon MF. The prediction of local recurrence in rectal adenocarcinoma by histopathological examination. Int J Colorectal Dis 1988;3(2):127–31.
23. Wiggers T, van de Velde CJ. The circumferential margin in rectal cancer. Recommendations based on the Dutch Total Mesorectal Excision Study. Eur J Cancer 2002;38(7):973–6.
24. Nagtegaal ID, van de Velde CJ, van der Worp E, et al. Macroscopic evaluation of rectal cancer resection specimen: clinical significance of the pathologist in quality control. J Clin Oncol 2002;20(7):1729–34.
25. Enker WE, Levi GS. Macroscopic assessment of mesorectal excision. Cancer 2009;115(21):4890–4.
26. Quirke P, Steele R, Monson J, et al. Effect of the plane of surgery achieved on local recurrence in patients with operable rectal cancer: a prospective study

using data from the MRC CR07 and NCIC-CTG CO16 randomised clinical trial. Lancet 2009;373(9666):821–8.

27. Nagtegaal ID, Quirke P. What is the role for the circumferential margin in the modern treatment of rectal cancer? J Clin Oncol 2008;26(2):303–12.

28. Adam IJ, Mohamdee MO, Martin IG, et al. Role of circumferential margin involvement in the local recurrence of rectal cancer. Lancet 1994;344(8924):707–11.

29. Birbeck KF, Macklin CP, Tiffin NJ, et al. Rates of circumferential resection margin involvement vary between surgeons and predict outcomes in rectal cancer surgery. Ann Surg 2002;235(4):449–57.

30. Poon JT, Law WL. Laparoscopic resection for rectal cancer: a review. Ann Surg Oncol 2009;16:3038–47.

31. Zhou ZG, Hu M, Li Y, et al. Laparoscopic versus open total mesorectal excision with anal sphincter preservation for low rectal cancer. Surg Endosc 2004;18(8): 1211–5.

32. Heald RJ, Moran BJ, Ryall RD, et al. Rectal cancer: the Basingstoke experience of total mesorectal excision, 1978–1997. Arch Surg 1998;133(8):894–9.

33. Cecil TD, Sexton R, Moran BJ, et al. Total mesorectal excision results in low local recurrence rates in lymph node-positive rectal cancer. Dis Colon Rectum 2004; 47(7):1145–9 [discussion: 1149–50].

34. Gouvas N, Tsiaoussis J, Pechlivanides G, et al. Quality of surgery for rectal carcinoma: comparison between open and laparoscopic approaches. Am J Surg 2009;198(5):702–8.

35. Bretagnol F, Lelong B, Laurent C, et al. The oncological safety of laparoscopic total mesorectal excision with sphincter preservation for rectal carcinoma. Surg Endosc 2005;19(7):892–6.

36. Law WL, Lee YM, Choi HK, et al. Laparoscopic and open anterior resection for upper and mid rectal cancer: an evaluation of outcomes. Dis Colon Rectum 2006;49(8):1108–15.

37. Morino M, Allaix ME, Giraudo G, et al. Laparoscopic versus open surgery for extraperitoneal rectal cancer: a prospective comparative study. Surg Endosc 2005;19(11):1460–7.

38. Strohlein MA, Grutzner KU, Jauch KW, et al. Comparison of laparoscopic vs. open access surgery in patients with rectal cancer: a prospective analysis. Dis Colon Rectum 2008;51(4):385–91.

39. Havenga K, Enker WE, McDermott K, et al. Male and female sexual and urinary function after total mesorectal excision with autonomic nerve preservation for carcinoma of the rectum. J Am Coll Surg 1996;182(6):495–502.

40. Jayne DG, Brown JM, Thorpe H, et al. Bladder and sexual function following resection for rectal cancer in a randomized clinical trial of laparoscopic versus open technique. Br J Surg 2005;92(9):1124–32.

41. Masui H, Ike H, Yamaguchi S, et al. Male sexual function after autonomic nerve-preserving operation for rectal cancer. Dis Colon Rectum 1996;39(10): 1140–5.

42. Liang JT, Lai HS, Lee PH. Laparoscopic pelvic autonomic nerve-preserving surgery for patients with lower rectal cancer after chemoradiation therapy. Ann Surg Oncol 2007;14(4):1285–7.

43. Asoglu O, Matlim T, Karanlik H, et al. Impact of laparoscopic surgery on bladder and sexual function after total mesorectal excision for rectal cancer. Surg Endosc 2009;23(2):296–303.

44. Jones OM, Stevenson AR, Stitz RW, et al. Preservation of sexual and bladder function after laparoscopic rectal surgery. Colorectal Dis 2009;11(5):489–95.

45. Buunen M, Bonjer HJ, Hop WC, et al. COLOR II. A randomized clinical trial comparing laparoscopic and open surgery for rectal cancer. Dan Med Bull 2009;56(2):89–91.
46. Kitano S, Inomata M, Sato A, et al. Randomized controlled trial to evaluate laparoscopic surgery for colorectal cancer: Japan Clinical Oncology Group Study JCOG 0404. Jpn J Clin Oncol 2005;35(8):475–7.
47. Fleshman J. American College of Surgeons Oncology Group (ACOSOG)-Z6051. A Phase III prospective randomized trial comparing laparoscopic-assisted resection versus open resection for rectal cancer. Available at: http://clinicaltrials.gov/ct2/show/NCT00726622. Accessed March 18, 2010.
48. Available at: http://clinicaltrials.gov/ct2/show/NCT00470951?cond=%22Rectal+Neoplasms%22&rank=41. Accessed March 20, 2010.
49. Available at: http://clinicaltrials.gov/ct2/show/NCT00007930?cond=%22Rectal+Neoplasms%22&rank=121. Accessed March 20, 2010.
50. Available at: http://www.fascrs.org/physicians/position_statements/laparoscopic_proctectomy/. Accessed August 21, 2010.
51. Marcello PW, Fleshman JW, Milsom JW, et al. Hand-assisted laparoscopic vs. laparoscopic colorectal surgery: a multicenter, prospective, randomized trial. Dis Colon Rectum 2008;51(6):818–26 [discussion: 826–8].
52. Aalbers AG, Biere SS, van Berge Henegouwen MI, et al. Hand-assisted or laparoscopic-assisted approach in colorectal surgery: a systematic review and meta-analysis. Surg Endosc 2008;22(8):1769–80.
53. Available at: http://clinicaltrials.gov/ct2/show/NCT00651677?term=hand+AND+rectal+cancer&rank=1. Accessed March 20, 2010.
54. Baik SH, Kwon HY, Kim JS, et al. Robotic versus laparoscopic low anterior resection of rectal cancer: short-term outcome of a prospective comparative study. Ann Surg Oncol 2009;16(6):1480–7.
55. Baik SH, Ko YT, Kang CM, et al. Robotic tumor-specific mesorectal excision of rectal cancer: short-term outcome of a pilot randomized trial. Surg Endosc 2008;22(7):1601–8.
56. Patriti A, Ceccarelli G, Bartoli A, et al. Short- and medium-term outcome of robot-assisted and traditional laparoscopic rectal resection. JSLS 2009;13(2):176–83.
57. Berguer R, Smith W. An ergonomic comparison of robotic and laparoscopic technique: the influence of surgeon experience and task complexity. J Surg Res 2006;134(1):87–92.
58. Senagore AJ, Luchtefeld MA, Mackeigan JM. What is the learning curve for laparoscopic colectomy? Am Surg 1995;61(8):681–5.
59. Simons AJ, Anthone GJ, Ortega AE, et al. Laparoscopic-assisted colectomy learning curve. Dis Colon Rectum 1995;38(6):600–3.
60. Wishner JD, Baker JW Jr, Hoffman GC, et al. Laparoscopic-assisted colectomy. The learning curve. Surg Endosc 1995;9(11):1179–83.
61. The American Society of Colon and Rectal Surgeons approved statement: laparoscopic colectomy for curable cancer. Surg Endosc 2004;18(8):A1.
62. Park IJ, Choi GS, Lim KH, et al. Multidimensional analysis of the learning curve for laparoscopic resection in rectal cancer. J Gastrointest Surg 2009;13(2):275–81.
63. Ross HM, Simmang CL, Fleshman JW, et al. Adoption of laparoscopic colectomy: results and implications of ASCRS hands-on course participation. Surg Innov 2008;15(3):179–83.

Chemoradiation for Rectal Cancer: Rationale, Approaches, and Controversies

Bruce D. Minsky, MD

KEYWORDS

• Chemoradiation • Rectal cancer • Radiation

The standard treatment of T3 and/or N+ rectal cancer is chemoradiation (CMT). When fluorouracil (5-FU) is used concurrently with CMT, continuous infusion (CI) is the standard.[1,2] As an alternative, capecitabine can be substituted for CI 5-FU. However, if the ongoing NSABP R-04 trial, which is comparing preoperative CMT with CI 5-FU with capecitabine (with or without oxaliplatin), reveals that capecitabine is inferior this approach would need to be reevaluated.

The regimen used for the adjuvant chemotherapy alone component of treatment is different. Based on the efficacy shown in patients with stage III colon cancer, the combination of CI 5-FU plus oxaliplatin (FOLFOX) has replaced CI 5-FU as a standard postoperative regimen.[3] Other agents such as irinotecan[4] and bevacizumab[5] have not improved survival in stage III colon cancer and therefore are not used in the adjuvant management of rectal cancer.

In contrast to adjuvant colon cancer in which 3-year and possibly 2-year[6] disease-free survival predicts for 5-year survival, the INT 0114 postoperative CMT rectal adjuvant trial showed that local control and survival continue to decrease beyond 5 years.[7] At 7 years local failure rate was 17% and the survival was 56% compared with 14% and 64%, respectively, at 5 years. Both surgeons and hospitals with higher volumes of rectal cancer surgery have improved outcomes compared with those with lower volumes.[8]

Two randomized trials of preoperative versus postoperative CMT for clinically resectable rectal cancer have been performed; NSABP R0-3[9] and the German CAO/ARO/AIO 94.[10] The German trial complete the planned accrual of more than 800 patients and randomized patients with uT3/4 and/or LN+ rectal cancers less

Department of Radiation and Cellular Oncology, University of Chicago Medical Center, 5841 South Maryland Avenue, MC-1000, Chicago, IL 60637, USA
E-mail address: bruce.minsky@uchospitals.edu

Surg Oncol Clin N Am 19 (2010) 803–818
doi:10.1016/j.soc.2010.06.001
surgonc.theclinics.com

than 16 cm from the anal verge to preoperative CMT (with CI 5-FU weeks 1 and 5) versus postoperative CMT.[10] Patients were stratified by surgeon and all underwent total mesorectal excision (TME). Compared with postoperative CMT, patients who received preoperative therapy had a significant decrease in local failure (6% vs 15%, $P = .006$), acute toxicity (27% vs 40%, $P = .001$), chronic toxicity (14% vs 24%, $P = .012$), and in those 194 patients judged by the surgeon before treatment to require an abdominoperineal resection (APR), a significant increase in sphincter preservation (39% vs 20%, $P = .004$). With a median follow-up of 40 months there was no difference in 5-year survival (74% vs 76%). A subsequent analysis revealed that the treatment center, schedule, and gender were independent prognostic factors for local control.[11]

The NSABP R-03 accrued only 267 of a planned 900 patients with cT3-4 rectal cancer.[9] Patients received induction chemotherapy followed by conventional CMT and were randomized to receive it either preoperatively or postoperatively. TME was not required and some patients underwent a local excision.

Compared with postoperative therapy, patients who received preoperative therapy had a significant improvement in 5-year disease-free survival (65% vs 53%, $P = .011$) and a borderline significant improvement in 5-year overall survival (75% vs 66%, $P = .065$). There was no difference in 5-year local recurrence (11%). There was a corresponding higher incidence of grade 4+ toxicity (33% vs 23%) but the incidence of grade 3+ toxicity was lower (41% vs 50%). Based on a prospective office assessment by the operating surgeon, there was no improvement in sphincter preservation (48% vs 39%).

The NSABP results are opposite to the German trial and are likely because only 267 of the 900 planned patients were accrued, thereby limiting the statistical power to detect differences. Therefore, based on the German CAO/ARO/AIO 94 randomized trial, most patients now receive preoperative CMT.

CLINICAL STAGING OF RECTAL CANCER

Transrectal ultrasound and high-resolution magnetic resonance imaging (MRI) are the most accurate tools in predicting T stage of rectal cancers. In the United States, ultrasound is used most commonly, whereas in many European countries high-resolution MRI is preferred. High-resolution MRI also allows for identification of patients likely to have close or positive radial margins if they underwent initial surgery and therefore are selected to receive preoperative therapy.[12]

The overall accuracy in predicting T stage is approximately 50% to 90% with ultrasound[13] or high-resolution MRI[14] and 50% to 70% with computed tomography (CT) or conventional MRI.[15] [^{18}F]Fluorodeoxyglucose (FDG)-positron emission tomography (PET) may be more accurate compared with CT for identification of metastatic disease.[16] The use of PET to restage patients following preoperative CMT remains controversial.[17-19]

Identification of positive lymph nodes is more difficult. The overall accuracy in detecting positive pelvic lymph nodes with the techniques outlined earlier is approximately 50% to 75%. The accuracy of MRI is similar to CT; however, it is improved with the use of external and/or endorectal coils. Both CT and MRI can identify lymph nodes measuring 1 cm or greater, although enlarged lymph nodes are not pathognomonic of tumor involvement. The accuracy of ultrasound for the detection of involved perirectal lymph nodes may be augmented if combined with fine needle aspiration.[20] Despite these advances, the ability to accurately predict the pathologic stage following preoperative CMT with MRI,[21,22] ultrasound,[23] FDG-PET[19] or physical examination[24] remains suboptimal.

After preoperative therapy overstaging is common, especially when there is a fibrotic thickening of the rectal wall. A high level of accuracy has been observed by phased array MRI for differentiating ypT0-2 versus ypT3.[25] Both diffusion-weighted MRI and FDG-PET have been used to monitor therapy response and to predict outcome to preoperative therapy. There is a decrease in standardized uptake value (SUV) on post-radiation FDG-PET in responders when compared with nonresponders, but the clinical value of this information remains to be determined.[26]

APPROACHES TO PREOPERATIVE THERAPY

There are 2 approaches to preoperative therapy. The first, used most commonly in Northern Europe and Scandinavia, is the short course (25 Gy in 5 fractions). In contrast, most other investigators recommend standard course (50.4 Gy in 28 fractions) combined with concurrent systemic chemotherapy (CMT). The primary reasons for this preference are the lack of sphincter preservation and the inability to safely combine adequate doses of systemic chemotherapy with short course radiation. CMT trials cannot be directly compared with short course radiation trials because they exclude patients with cT1-2 disease. Short course radiation trials include patients with cT1-3 disease.

Bujko and colleagues[27,28] performed a randomized trial of 2 preoperative approaches. A total of 316 patients with cT3 rectal cancer were randomized to short course radiation followed by surgery versus conventional preoperative CMT followed by surgery. All tumors were above the anorectal ring, TME was performed for distal tumors, and there was no radiation quality control review. There were no significant differences in local control or survival. The incidence of positive circumferential radial margins (CRM+) was lower following CMT compared with radiation alone (4% vs 13%, $P = .017$). Results from a similar Australian trial are pending.

IS POSTOPERATIVE ADJUVANT CHEMOTHERAPY NECESSARY?

Two randomized trials question whether postoperative chemotherapy is beneficial in patients with cT3 rectal cancer who receive preoperative therapy. The EORTC 22921 was a 4-arm randomized trial of 1011 patients who received preoperative 45 Gy with or without concurrent bolus 5-FU/leucovorin followed by surgery with or without 4 cycles of postoperative 5-FU/leucovorin.[29] Only 37% had a TME. The FFCD 9203 was a 2-arm randomized trial of 742 patients randomized to preoperative 45 Gy with or without bolus 5-FU/leucovorin.[30] However, all patients were scheduled to receive postoperative chemotherapy and 73% did receive it.

The EORTC trial revealed a significant decrease in the local failure rate in those patients who receive CMT compared with radiation (8% to 10% vs 17%, $P<.001$) but no difference in 5-year survival (65%). However, only 43% received 95% or more of the planned postoperative chemotherapy, which may explain the negative results. Furthermore, a subset analysis of the EORTC trial revealed that patients who responded to preoperative CMT had a survival benefit from postoperative chemotherapy.[31] The FFCD trial reported a similar decrease in local failure (8% vs 17%, $P<.05$), a corresponding increase in pathologic complete response rate (pCR) (11% vs 4%, $P<.05$), but no survival benefit (68% vs 67%) with preoperative CMT.

Given that most patients did not receive adequate doses of postoperative chemotherapy in the EORTC trial and the FFCD trial tested only the effect of 6 weeks of concurrent chemotherapy with preoperative radiation, preoperative CMT followed by surgery and 4 months of postoperative adjuvant chemotherapy (FOLFOX) remains the standard practice in North America. However, there remains considerable controversy in some European countries regarding its use.[32]

Most investigators believe the treatment is reasonable and use the same adjuvant chemotherapy for adjuvant colon and rectal cancer. For patients who receive preoperative CMT, and are selected to receive postoperative adjuvant chemotherapy, 4 months (8 cycles) of mFOLFOX6 is recommended.

CMT FOR NODE-NEGATIVE RECTAL CANCER

There may be a subset of patients with pT3N0 disease who may not require adjuvant therapy.[33,34] Patients who undergo a TME, have at least 12 nodes examined, and have stage pT3N0 disease likely do not need the radiation component of CMT. The approximately 3% to 4% benefit in local control with radiation may not be worth the risks, especially in women of reproductive age. However, patients with pT3N0 tumors with either adverse pathologic features, resected without a TME, or in whom fewer than 12 nodes have been examined should still receive postoperative CMT.

Neither MRI nor any other imaging modality or clinicopathologic factor can reproducibly identify patients with LN+ disease.[35] Tumor regression grade[36–38] may help predict LN+. The development of more accurate methods to identify LN+ disease, including imaging techniques and/or molecular markers, is essential because more patients are being treated with preoperative CMT.

In the German trial, 18% of patients clinically staged as cT3N0 preoperatively and who underwent initial surgery without preoperative therapy had pT1-2N0 disease. Therefore, those patients would have been overtreated if they had received preoperative therapy. Although not ideal, preoperative therapy is still preferred to performing surgery first because even after preoperative CMT (which downstages tumors) Guillem and colleagues[39] reported that 22% have ypN+ disease at the time of surgery. In patients who undergo surgery alone this number is as high as 40%.[40] These patients then require postoperative CMT, which, compared with preoperative CMT, has inferior local control, higher acute and chronic toxicity, and, if a low anastomosis is performed, inferior functional results. Furthermore, the incidence of positive nodes was not dependent on the distance from the anal verge.[39] Of the 103 patients with tumors from 0 to 5 cm from the anal verge, 23% were ypN+, whereas of the 85 patients with tumors 6 to 12 cm from the anal verge the incidence was 20%. These data suggest that up to 12 cm from the anal verge, the risk of positive nodes (and likely local recurrence) is similar.

DISTANCE FROM THE ANAL VERGE

There are no prospective randomized data examining the effect of the distance from the anal verge on local recurrence. The available data are subset analysis from randomized trials that were not stratified by distance. Additional variables could have contributed to the differences in local failure. For example, TME was used in the Dutch CVKO and German trials and not in the Swedish trial. All 3 trials included patients with tumors more than 12 cm from the anal verge in the upper or high category. Because the peritoneal reflection varies from 12 to 16 cm some patients with tumors above the peritoneal reflection (colon cancer) were included in the 3 trials. Most investigators now limit preoperative treatment to tumors less than 12 cm from the anal verge.[39] Distance measurements using a flexible proctoscope are less accurate than a straight proctoscope. Flexible scopes were used in the Dutch CKVO trial. The German trial used a straight scope. In the Swedish trial proctoscopic information was not mentioned. However, eligibility was limited to tumors "below the promontory as identified by barium enema." The Polish trial is not discussed because all tumors were within reach by digital examination.[27]

As seen in **Table 1**, by univariate analysis, high tumors in both the Dutch CKVO and Swedish trial (defined as >10.1 cm and 11 cm, respectively) had a lower incidence of local recurrence compared with mid and lower tumors. Short course radiation did not significantly decrease local recurrence. By multivariate analysis, tumor location was an independent prognostic variable in the Dutch trial. Radiation did significantly decrease local recurrence for mid tumors in both trials, whereas for lower tumors it was helpful only in the Swedish trial.

In contrast, there was no significant difference between mid and upper tumors in the German trial.[61] However, data were not provided. In a recent subset analysis, patients with tumors more than 6 cm had a lower local recurrence rate (Rodel, personal communication, 2009).

Given the conflicting data combined with the report from Guillem and colleagues confirming that the incidence of positive nodes (ypN0 disease following preoperative CMT) is the same from 0 to 12 cm from the anal verge, treatment decisions based on the current definitions of low versus mid versus high should not be used.

POSITIVE RADIAL (CIRCUMFERENTIAL) MARGINS

The radial (circumferential) margin also has a substantial effect on the local recurrence rate.[62] In the Dutch CKVO trial, 17% had positive circumferential margins. In a subset analysis by Nagtegaal and colleagues,[63] patients with positive circumferential margins who underwent TME alone had local recurrence rate of 17% after a low anterior resection and 30% after an APR. Few centers perform the necessary pathologic examination to detect positive circumferential margins.[64] High-resolution MRI can help identify patients who have positive margins as well as select those who may benefit from preoperative therapy.[65–67]

A positive circumferential margin following preoperative CMT is less favorable. Compared with 460 patients with negative circumferential margins, Baik and

Table 1
Effect of distance from the anal verge by univariate analysis

Location	Distance from the Anal Verge (cm)	Number	Surgery 5-year Local Failure (%)	Number	Preoperative Radiation Dose/ Fraction Size 5-year Local Failure (%)	P
Dutch CKVO						
High	≥10.1	271	6	262	4	Not significant
Middle	5.1–10	350	14	372	4	<0.001
Low	≤5	253	12	237	11	Not significant
Swedish Rectal Cancer Trial						
High	≥11	110	12	133	8	Not significant
Middle	6–10	198	26	185	9	<0.001
Low	≤5	146	27	136	10	0.003

colleagues[68] reported that the 44 patients with positive margins had a higher local recurrence (35% vs 11%) and decreased survival rates (27% vs 73%). An analysis of more than 17,500 pathologic specimens by Nagtegaal and Quirke[62] reported inferior survival in patients with CRM+ after neoadjuvant treatment compared with immediate surgery (hazard ratio [HR] 6.3; 95% confidence interval [CI], 3.7 to 16.7 vs HR 2.0; 95% CI, 1.4 to 2.9, respectively).

As reported with preoperative therapy, postoperative treatment has limited ability to control positive circumferential margins. In the MRC CR-07 trial, patients with positive radial margins who were selected to receive postoperative CMT had an 11% local recurrence rate.[69] Likewise, in a subset analysis of the Dutch CKVO trial, 50 Gy postoperatively did not compensate for positive margins.[70]

IS RADICAL SURGERY NECESSARY FOLLOWING PREOPERATIVE CMT?

One series has questioned the value of radical surgery in patients who had a biopsy-proven complete response.[71] However, it included patients with cT1-3 disease and has not been reproduced by other investigators. In series limited to patients with cT3 disease who received preoperative CMT, radical surgery is still necessary to fully evaluate if a pathologic response has been achieved. Neither posttreatment ultrasound[23,72] nor physical examination[73] is sufficient. The use of PET scan[19] and diffusion MRI[74] as noninvasive measures of response is being investigated and has reported mixed results. Although Kalff and colleagues[18] reported FDG-PET identification of residual viable tumor in 63 patients following CMT had a high positive predictive value (0.94; 95% CI 85%–99%), other groups have reported opposite results.

Glynne-Jones and colleagues[75] reviewed 218 phase II and 28 phase III trials of preoperative radiation or CMT and confirmed that clinical and/or radiologic response does not sufficiently correlate with pathologic response, and these investigators do not recommend a wait-and-see approach to surgery following preoperative therapy.

Experience with preoperative CMT followed by local excision is more limited. Most series select patients with cT3 disease who were either medically inoperable or refused radical surgery. Local recurrence rates range from 0% to 20% and 5-year survival ranges from 78% to 90%. Borschitz and colleagues[76] reported local recurrence rates by pathologic stage: ypT1: 2%, ypT2; 6% to 20%. Rates were as high as 43% in ypT3 tumors that did not respond to CMT. This approach is being prospectively tested in the ACOSOG 06031 trial. In this phase II trial, patients with uT2N0 disease received preoperative capecitabine + oxaliplatin (CAPOX) and radiation therapy. If following local excision they have stage ypT0-2 with negative margins they undergo observation only. If the postoperative stage is ypT3 or if the margins are positive then patients undergo radical surgery. A similar trial in France (GRECCAR 2) is designed to accrue 300 patients with cT2-3 disease.

CMT REGIMENS

Both cytotoxic and targeted chemotherapeutic agents have been incorporated into phase I/II combined modality programs, most commonly in the preoperative setting. Selected series are seen in **Table 2**. Most of the regimens reveal higher pCR rates compared with 5-FU alone (10% in the German trial). However, for some agents, with this increased pCR rate is an associated increase in acute toxicity.

However, 2 phase III trials have reported significantly higher acute toxicity with no benefit in the pCR rate with the addition of oxaliplatin to CI 5-FU–based CMT in patients with cT3-4 and/N+ rectal cancer. The STAR-01 trial randomized 747 patients to preoperative CMT with 50.4 Gy + CI 5-FU ± oxaliplatin (60 mg/m^2 weekly).[59] There was a significant increase in grade 3+ with oxaliplatin (24% vs 8%, $P<.001$) with no improvement in the pCR rate (15% vs 16%). The ACCORD trial randomized 598 patients to preoperative CMT with 50 Gy plus CAPOX versus 45 Gy plus capecitibine.[60] There was a similar significant increase in grade 3+ with oxaliplatin (25% vs 11%, $P<.001$) with no improvement in the pCR rate (19% vs 14%). Although local control and survival outcomes are pending, these early results underscore the importance of phase III data.

A similar question is being addressed in 3 ongoing phase III trials. In the United States the NSABP R-04 trial is a 4-arm trial (2 × 2 comparison) of CI 5-FU versus capecitabine-based preoperative CMT (50.4 Gy) with or without oxaliplatin. The CAO/ARO/AIO-04 and the PETACC-6 are 2-arm trials randomizing patients to preoperative 45 to 50.4 Gy + CI 5-FU (CAO/ARO/AIO-04) or capecitabine (PETACC-6) with or without oxaliplatin, added in the experimental arms of both studies to concomitant preoperative radiation as well as to postoperative 5-FU/capecitabine chemotherapy.

The role of targeted biologic agents such as bevacizumab is being tested. Preliminary phase I trials using preoperative CMT with CAPOX + bevacizumab reveal pCR rates of 18% to 24%.[44,77]

Although the report from Heidelberg with CAPEIRI reported a pCR rate of 25%[45] other trials with 5-FU, capecitabine, or CAPOX have more limited rates of 5% to 12%.[50,78] Whether the benefit of patient selection based on wild versus mutated KRAS seen in patients with metastatic disease is helpful in the adjuvant rectal setting is unknown.[77]

INDUCTION CHEMOTHERAPY

Chau and colleagues[55] have examined the use of induction CAPOX followed by CMT with capecitibine. This approach circumvents the need for the 4 months of postoperative chemotherapy. This pilot trial of 77 patients reported a 24% pCR rate. Because there is a 6-month interval between diagnosis and surgery the radiologic response rate was followed by MRI. After induction CAPOX the overall response rate was 88%, which increased to 97% following the completion of CMT, suggesting that there was no detriment in response rates. Based on these encouraging results the Spanish GCR-3 randomized phase II trial was developed comparing this approach with conventional preoperative CMT followed by surgery and postoperative chemotherapy.[57] A total of 108 patients received preoperative 50.4 Gy plus CAPOX and were randomized to receive 4 months of CAPOX either by induction or adjuvant (postoperative). Although the pCR rates were not different (14% vs 13%) both grade 3+ toxicity was lower (17% vs 51%, $P = .00004$) and the ability to receive all 4 chemotherapy cycles was higher (93% vs 51%, $P = .0001$) with the induction approach.

TUMOR RESPONSE

Although some series show no correlation,[79] most series suggest that there is improved outcome with increasing pathologic response to preoperative CMT.[80,81] A retrospective review of 566 patients who achieved a pCR after receiving a variety of preoperative CMT regimens at multiple European centers was reported by Capirci and colleagues.[82] With a median follow-up of 46 months the local recurrence rate was only 1.6% and the 5-year disease-free and overall survival were 85% and 90%, respectively.

Analysis of biopsies examining selected molecular markers[83–85] have had varying success in helping to select patients who may best respond to preoperative therapy. In a recent review, Kuremsky and colleagues[86] identified 1204 articles examining

Table 2
Selected novel preoperative CMT regimens

Author/Regimen	Number	Phase	RT (Gy)	pCR (%)	LF (%)	Gr 3 + Acute Toxicity[a]
Hofheinz et al,[41] CAPIRI	19	I	50.4/1.8	21	—	8% fatigue
Fakih et al,[42] CAPOX	12	I	50.4/1.8	27	—	—
Allal et al,[43] Irinotecan	37	I/II	50/1.25 twice daily	17	5 (3-y)	6% heme, infection, 24% GI, 15% skin
Willett et al,[44] CAPOX + bevicizumab	32	I/II	50.4/1.8	16	100 (5-y)	22% diarrhea, 9% HTN, 6% skin, 3% dehydration, abscess, pain, neuro
Das et al,[45] Capecitibine CI 5-FU (match pair analysis)	89 89	II	52.5/1.8 52.5/1.8	21 12	6 (3-y) 1 (3-y)	6% 6%
Hospers et al,[46] CAPOX	21	II	50.4/1.8	10	—	18% diarrhea
Machiels et al,[47] CAPOX	40	II	45/1.8	14	0 (14 M)	30% diarrhea, 5% vomiting, neutropenia, fever, fatigue, pain
Avallone et al,[48] FOLFOX/raltitrexed	31	II	45/1.5	42	0 (29 mo)	3% stomatitis, 22% diarrhea, 39% neutropenia
Ryan et al,[49] (CALGB 89901) FOLFOX	26	II	50.4/1.8	25	—	38% diarrhea, 19% fatigue
Rodel et al,[50] CAPOX + cetuximab	48	II	50.4/1.8	9	—	19% diarrhea
Krishnan et al,[51] Capecitabine	54	II	52.2/1.8	18	—	9% skin, 2% diarrhea
Crane et al,[52] Capecitabine + bevacizumab	25	II	50.5/1.8	32	7% 2-y	3% wound comp require surgery, 4% rash, 4% neuropathy

Study	No. of patients	Phase	RT dose/fraction	pCR (%)	Grade 3+ toxicity[a]	
Bertolini et al,[53] Induction cetuximab	40	II	50–50.4/1.8–2	8	—	15%
Navarro et al,[54] FOLFIRI	74	II	45/1.8	14	—	7% neutropenia, 14% diarrhea, 9% asthenia, 16% rectal/abdominal pain
Chau et al,[55] Induction CAPOX Capecitibine	77	II	50.4/1.8	24	—	7% heme, 4% GI, 3% GU, 43% skin
Mohiuddin et al,[56] (RTOG 0012) FOLFIRI CI 5-FU	54 / 52	II R	50.4–54/1.8 / 55.2–60/1.2 Twice daily	28 / 28	— / —	57% heme and nonheme / 51% heme and nonheme
Fernandez-Martos et al,[57] Induction CAPOX Postoperative CAPOX	56 / 52	II R	50.4/1.8	14 / 13	— / —	17% (P = .00004) / 51%
Valentini et al,[58] Oxaliplatin/raltitrexed 5-FU/CDDP	81 / 83	II R	50.4/1.8 / 50.4/1.8	36 / 24	— / —	16% / 7%
Aschele et al,[59] (STAR) CI 5-FU FOLFOX	295 / 291	III	50.3/1.8 / 50.4/1.8	16 / 15	— / —	15 (P<.001) / 24
Gerard et al,[60] (ACCORD) Capecitibine CAPEOX	379 / 368	III	45/1.8 / 50/1.8	14 / 19	— / —	11 (P<.001) / 25

Abbreviations: GI, gastrointestinal; GU, genitourinary; HTN, hypertension; LF, local failure; pCR, pathologic complete response rate; R, randomized phase II trial; RT, radiation dose/fraction size.

[a] Grade 3+ toxicity at the phase II (recommended dose) if available.

a total of 36 molecular biomarkers that may have predictive value. Restricting the analysis to patients treated with preoperative CMT and to gene products examined by 5 or more studies, only p53, epidermal growth factor receptor (EGFR), thymidylate synthase, Ki-67, p21, and bax/bcl-2 met these criteria. Of these products, quantitatively evaluated EGFR or EGFR polymorphisms, thymidylate synthase polymorphisms, and p21 have been identified as promising candidates that should be evaluated in larger prospective trials for their ability to guide preoperative therapy. Because the studies are limited retrospective trials and most did not examine multiple markers, the need for adjuvant therapy should still be based solely on T and N stage.

Konski and colleagues[87] performed pre- and posttreatment FDG-PET scans on 53 patients receiving preoperative CMT. By multivariate analysis the percent decrease in SUV was marginally trended in predicting pCR ($P = .07$).

RADIATION TECHNIQUES AND DOSE

The clinical usefulness of routine three-dimensional (3D) and intensity-modulated radiation therapy (IMRT) treatment planning techniques is being investigated.[88,89] The most important contribution of 3D treatment planning is the ability to plan and localize the target and normal tissues at all levels of the treatment volume and to obtain dose volume histogram data. An analysis of 3D treatment planning techniques at the Massachusetts General Hospital suggests that the volume of small bowel in the radiation field is decreased with protons compared with photons.[90] IMRT treatment planning techniques can further decrease the volume of small bowel in the field.[91] However, the clinical benefit of IMRT compared with 3D or conventional treatment delivery remains to be determined.[88] Guidelines for the definition and delineation of the clinical target volumes are available from several investigators.[92,93]

The RTOG R-0012 phase II randomized trial compared twice-daily preoperative CMT up to 60 Gy (1.2 Gy to 45.6 Gy, with a boost of 9.6–14.4 Gy) with conventional fractionation (1.8 Gy to 45 Gy, with a boost of 5.4–9.0 Gy) plus 5-FU/irinotecan.[56] Both regimens resulted in a 28% pCR rate, but were also associated with a greater than 40% rate of grade 3 to 4 acute toxicity.

SUMMARY

Many controversies remain. For example, should patients receive short course radiation or CMT? Will delayed surgery after short course radiation improve downstaging? Is postoperative adjuvant chemotherapy necessary for all patients and should the type of surgery following CMT be based on the response rate? Can we develop more accurate imaging techniques and/or molecular markers to identify patients with positive pelvic nodes to reduce the chance of overtreatment with preoperative therapy? Will more effective systemic agents both improve the results of CMT as well as modify the need for pelvic radiation? These questions and others remain active areas of clinical investigation.

REFERENCES

1. Krook JE, Moertel CG, Gunderson LL, et al. Effective surgical adjuvant therapy for high-risk rectal carcinoma. N Engl J Med 1991;324:709–15.
2. Twelves C, Wong A, Nowacki MP, et al. Capecitabine as adjuvant treatment for stage III colon cancer. N Engl J Med 2005;352:2696–704.
3. Andre T, Boni C, Mounedji-Boudiaf L, et al. Oxaliplatin, fluorouracil, and leucovorin as adjuvant treatment for colon cancer. N Engl J Med 2004;350:2343–51.

4. Saltz LB, Niedzwiecki D, Hollis D, et al. Irinotecan fluorouracil plus leucovorin is not superior to fluorouracil plus leucovorin alone as adjuvant treatment for stage III colon cancer: results of CALGB 89803. J Clin Oncol 2007;25:3456–61.
5. Wolmark N, Yothers G, O'Connell MJ, et al. A phase III trial comparing mFOLFOX6 plus bevacizumab in stage II or III carcinoma of the colon: results of NSABP protocol C-08. Proc ASCO 2009;27:793s.
6. Sargent D, Yothers G, van Cutsem E, et al. Use of two-year disease-free survival (DFS) as a primary endpoint in stage III adjuvant colon cancer trials with fluoro-pyrimidines with or without oxaliplatin or irinotecan: new data from 12,676 patients from MOSAIC, X-ACT, PETACC-3, NSABP C-06 and C-07, and C89803. Proc ASCO 2009;27:170s.
7. Tepper JE, O'Connell MJ, Niedzwiecki D, et al. Adjuvant therapy in rectal cancer: analysis of stage, sex, and local control – final report of Intergroup 0114. J Clin Oncol 2002;20:1744–50.
8. Meyerhardt JA, Tepper JE, Neidzwiecki D, et al. Impact of hospital procedure volume on surgical operation and long-term outcomes in high risk curatively re-sected rectal cancer: findings from the Intergroup 0114 study. J Clin Oncol 2004;22:166–74.
9. Roh MS, Colangelo LH, O'Connell MJ, et al. Pre-operative multimodality therapy improves disease-free survival in patients with carcinoma of the rectum (NSABP-R-03). J Clin Oncol 2009;27:5124–30.
10. Sauer R, Becker H, Hohenberger P, et al. Preoperative chemoradiotherapy as compared with postoperative chemoradiotherapy for locally advanced rectal cancer. N Engl J Med 2004;351:11–20.
11. Fietkau R, Rodel C, Hohenberger W, et al. Rectal cancer delivery of radio-therapy in adequate time and with adequate dose is influenced by treatment center, treatment schedule, and gender and is prognostic parameter for local control: results of study CAO/ARO/AIO-94. Int J Radiat Oncol Biol Phys 2007;67:1008–19.
12. Salerno GV, Daniels IR, Moran BJ, et al. Magnetic resonance imaging prediction of an involved surgical resection margin in low rectal cancer. Dis Colon Rectum 2009;52:632–9.
13. Barbaro B, Valentini V, Coco C, et al. Tumor vascularity evaluated by transrectal color doppler US in predicting therapy outcome for low-lying rectal cancer. Int J Radiat Oncol Biol Phys 2005;63:1304–8.
14. Valentini V, DePaoli A, Gambacorta MA, et al. Chemoradiation with infusional 5-FU and ZD1839 (Gefitinib - Iressa) in patients with locally advanced rectal cancer: a phase II trial. Int J Radiat Oncol Biol Phys 2006;66:s168.
15. Kim NK, Kim MJ, Park JK, et al. Preoperative staging of rectal cancer with MRI: accuracy and clinical usefulness. Ann Surg Oncol 2000;7:732–7.
16. Nahas CS, Akhurst T, Yeung H, et al. Positron emission tomography detection of distant metastatic or synchronous disease in patients with locally advanced rectal cancer receiving preoperative chemoradiation. Ann Surg Oncol 2008;15:704–11.
17. Dietz DW, Dehdashti F, Grigsby PW, et al. Tumor hypoxia detected by positron emission tomography with 60Cu-ATSM as a predictor of response and survival in patients undergoing neoadjuvant chemoradiotherapy for rectal carcinoma: a pilot study. Dis Colon Rectum 2008;51:1641–8.
18. Kalff V, Ware R, Heriot A, et al. Radiation changes do not interfere with postche-moradiation restaging of patients with rectal cancer by FDG PET/CT before cura-tive surgical therapy. Int J Radiat Oncol Biol Phys 2009;74:60–6.

19. Kristiansen C, Loft A, Berthelsen AK, et al. PET/CT and histopathologic response to preoperative chemoradiation therapy in locally advanced rectal cancer. Dis Colon Rectum 2008;51:21–5.

20. Shami VM, Parmer KS, Waxman I. Clinical impact of endoscopic ultrasound and endoscopic ultrasound-guided fine-needle aspiration in the management of rectal carcinoma. Dis Colon Rectum 2004;47:59–65.

21. Kim YH, Kim DY, Kim TH, et al. Usefulness of magnetic resonance volumetric evaluation in predicting response to preoperative concurrent chemoradiotherapy in patients with resectable rectal cancer. Int J Radiat Oncol Biol Phys 2005;62:761–8.

22. Kuo LJ, Chern MC, Tsou MH, et al. Interpretation of magnetic resonance imaging for locally advanced rectal carcinoma after preoperative chemoradiation therapy. Dis Colon Rectum 2005;48:23–8.

23. Barbaro B, Schulsinger A, Valentini V, et al. The accuracy of transrectal ultrasound in predicting the pathological stage of low-lying rectal cancer after preoperative chemoradiation therapy. Int J Radiat Oncol Biol Phys 1999;43:1043–7.

24. Guillem JG, Chessin DB, Shia J, et al. Clinical examination following preoperative chemoradiation for rectal cancer is not a reliable surrogate endpoint. J Clin Oncol 2005;23:3475–9.

25. Barbaro B, Fiorucci C, Tebala C, et al. Locally advanced rectal cancer: MR imaging in prediction of response after preoperative chemotherapy and radiation therapy. Radiology 2009;250:730–9.

26. Calvo FA, Domper M, Matute R, et al. 18F-FDG positron emission tomography staging and restaging in rectal cancer treated with preoperative chemoradiation. Int J Radiat Oncol Biol Phys 2004;58:528–35.

27. Bujko K, Nowacki MP, Nasierowska-Guttmejer A, et al. Long term results of a randomized trial comparing preoperative short-course radiotherapy with preoperative conventionally fractionated chemoradiation for rectal cancer. Br J Surg 2006;93:1215–23.

28. Bujko K, Nowacki MP, Nasierowska-Guttmejer A, et al. Sphincter preservation following preoperative radiotherapy for rectal cancer: report of a randomized trial comparing short-term radiotherapy vs. conventionally fractionated radiochemotherapy. Radiother Oncol 2004;72:15–24.

29. Bosset JF, Collette L, Bardet E, et al. Chemotherapy with preoperative radiotherapy in rectal cancer. N Engl J Med 2006;355:1114–23.

30. Gerard JP, Conroy T, Bonnetain F. Preoperative radiotherapy with or without concurrent fluorouracil and leucovorin in T3-4 rectal cancers: results of FFCD 9203. J Clin Oncol 2006;28:4620–5.

31. Collette L, Bosset JF, den Dulk M, et al. Patients with curative resection of cT3-4 rectal cancer after preoperative radiotherapy or radiochemotherapy: does anybody benefit from adjuvant fluorouracil-based chemotherapy? A trial of the European Organisation for Research and Treatment of Cancer Radiation Oncology Group. J Clin Oncol 2007;25:4379–86.

32. Valentini V, Aristei C, Glimelius B, et al. Multidisciplinary rectal cancer management: 2nd European Rectal Cancer Consensus Conference. Radiother Oncol 2009;92:148–63.

33. Green FL, Stewart AK, Norton HJ. New tumor-node-metastasis staging system for node-positive (stage III) rectal cancer: an analysis. J Clin Oncol 2004;22:1778–84.

34. Nissan A, Stojadinovic A, Shia J, et al. Predictors of recurrence in patients with T2 and early T3, N0 adenocarcinoma of the rectum treated with surgery alone. J Clin Oncol 2006;24:4078–84.

35. Kim JH, Beets GL, Kim MJ, et al. High-resolution MR imaging for nodal staging in rectal cancer: are there any criteria in addition to the size? Eur J Radiol 2004;52: 78–83.
36. Read TE, Andujar JE, Caushaj FP, et al. Neoadjuvant therapy for rectal cancer: histologic response of the primary tumor predicts nodal status. Dis Colon Rectum 2004;47:825–31.
37. Roedel C, Fietkau R, Raab R, et al. Tumor regression grading as a prognostic factor in patients with locally advanced rectal cancer treated with preoperative radiochemotherapy. Int J Radiat Oncol Biol Phys 2004;140:60s.
38. Vecchio FM, Valentini V, Minsky B, et al. The relationship of pathologic tumor regression grade (TRG) and outcome after preoperative therapy in rectal cancer. Int J Radiat Oncol Biol Phys 2005;62:752–60.
39. Guillem JG, Diaz-Gonzalez J, Minsky BD, et al. cT3N0 rectal cancer: potential overtreatment with preoperative chemoradiotherapy is warranted. J Clin Oncol 2008;26:368–73.
40. Mendenhall WM, Bland KI, Rout WR, et al. Clinically resectable adenocarcinoma of the rectum treated with preoperative irradiation and surgery. Dis Colon Rectum 1988;31:287–90.
41. Hofheinz RD, von Gerstenberg-Helldorf B, Wenz F, et al. Phase I trial of capecitabine and weekly irinotecan in combination with radiotherapy for neoadjuvant therapy of rectal cancer. J Clin Oncol 2005;23:1350–7.
42. Fakih MG, Rajput A, Yang GY, et al. A phase I study of weekly intravenous oxaliplatin in combination with oral daily capecitabine and radiation therapy in the neoadjuvant treatment of rectal adenocarcinoma. Int J Radiat Oncol Biol Phys 2006;65:1462–70.
43. Allal A, Bieri S, Gervaz P, et al. Preoperative concomitant hyperfractionated radiotherapy and gemcitaibine for locally advanced rectal cancers: a phase I-II trial. Cancer J 2005;11:133–9.
44. Willett CG, Duda D, di Tomaso E, et al. Efficacy, safety, and biomarkers of neoadjuvant bevacizumab, radiation therapy, and fluorouracil in rectal cancer: a multidisciplinary phase II study. J Clin Oncol 2009;27:3020–6.
45. Das P, Lin EH, Bhatia S, et al. Preoperative chemoradiotherapy with capecitabine versus protracted infusion 5-fluorouracil for rectal cancer: a matched-pair analysis. Int J Radiat Oncol Biol Phys 2006;66:1378–83.
46. Hospers GA, Punt CJ, Tesselaar ME, et al. Preoperative chemoradiotherapy with capecitabine and oxaliplatin in locally advanced rectal cancer: a phase I-II multicenter study of the Dutch Colorectal Cancer Group. Ann Surg Oncol 2007;14: 2773–9.
47. Machiels JP, Duck L, Honhon B, et al. Phase II study of preoperative oxaliplatin, capecitabine, and external beam radiotherapy in patients with rectal cancer: the RadiOxCape study. Ann Oncol 2005;16:1898–905.
48. Avallone A, Delrio P, Guida C, et al. Biweekly oxaliplatin, raltitrexed, 5-fluorouracil and folinic acid combination chemotherapy during preoperative radiation therapy for locally advanced rectal cancer: a phase I-II study. Br J Cancer 2006;94:1809–15.
49. Ryan DP, Niedzwiecki D, Hollis D, et al. Phase I/II study of preoperative oxaliplatin, fluorouracil, and external-beam radiation therapy in patients with locally advanced rectal cancer: Cancer and Leukemia Group B 89901. J Clin Oncol 2006;24:2557–62.
50. Rodel C, Arnold D, Hipp M, et al. Phase I-II trial of cetuximab, capecitabine, oxaliplatin, and radiotherapy as preoperative treatment in rectal cancer. Int J Radiat Oncol Biol Phys 2008;70:1081–6.

51. Krishnan S, Janjan NA, Hoff PM, et al. Phase II study of capecitabine (Xeloda) and concomitant boost radiotherapy in patients with locally advanced rectal cancer. Int J Radiat Oncol Biol Phys 2006;66:762–71.

52. Crane CH, Eng C, Feig BW, et al. Phase II trial of neoadjuvant bevacizumab (BEV), capecitabine (CAP), and radiotherapy (XRT) for locally advanced rectal cancer. Proc ASCO 2008;26:200s.

53. Bertolini F, Chiara S, Bengala C, et al. Neoadjuvant treatment with single-agent cetuximab followed by 5-FU, cetuximab, and pelvic radiotherapy: a phase II study in locally advanced rectal cancer. Int J Radiat Oncol Biol Phys 2009;73:466–72.

54. Navarro M, Dotor E, Rivera F, et al. A phase II study of preoperative radiotherapy and concomitant weekly irinotecan in combination with protracted venous infusion 5-fluorouracil for resectable locally advanced rectal cancer. Int J Radiat Oncol Biol Phys 2006;66:201–5.

55. Chau I, Brown G, Cunningham D, et al. Neoadjuvant capecitabine and oxaliplatin followed by synchronous chemoradiation and total mesorectal excision in magnetic resonance imaging defined poor risk rectal cancer. J Clin Oncol 2006;24:668–74.

56. Mohiuddin M, Winter K, Mitchell E, et al. Randomized phase II study of neoadjuvant combined modality chemoradiation for distal rectal cancer: Radiation Therapy Oncology Group Trial 0012. J Clin Oncol 2006;24:650–5.

57. Fernandez-Martos C, Aparicio J, Salud A, et al. Multicenter randomized phase II study of chemoradiation (CRT) followed by surgery (S) and chemotherapy (CT) versus induction chemotherapy followed by CRT and S in high-risk rectal cancer: GCR-3 final efficacy and safety results. Proc ASCO 2009;27:4103.

58. Valentini V, Coco C, Minsky BD, et al. Randomized multicenter phase IIB study of preoperative chemoradiotherapy in T3 mid-distal recta cancer: raltitrexed + oxaliplatin + radiotherapy versus cisplatin + 5-fluorouracil + radiotherapy. Int J Radiat Oncol Biol Phys 2008;70:403–12.

59. Aschele C, Pinto C, Cordio S, et al. Preoperative fluorouracil (FU) based chemoradiation with and without weekly oxaliplatin in locally advanced rectal cancer: pathologic response analysis of the Studio Terapia Adjuvante Retto (STAR)-01 randomized phase III trial. Proc ASCO 2009;27:804s.

60. Gerard JP, Azria D, Gourgou-Bourgade S, et al. Randomized multicenter phase III trial comparing two neoadjuvant chemoradiotherapy (CT-RT) regimens (RT45-Cap versus RT50-Capox) in patients with locally advanced rectal cancer (LARC): results of the ACCORD 12/0405 PRODIGE 2. Proc ASCO 2009;27:797s.

61. Sauer R, Roedel C. The author's reply. N Engl J Med 2005;352:510–1.

62. Nagtegaal ID, Quirke P. What is the role for the circumferential margin in the modern treatment of rectal cancer? J Clin Oncol 2008;26:303–12.

63. Nagtegaal ID, van de Velde CJ, Marijnen CA, et al. Low rectal cancer: a call for a change of approach in abdominoperineal resection. J Clin Oncol 2005;23:9257–64.

64. Guillem JG, Chessin DB, Shia J, et al. A prospective pathologic analysis using whole mount sections of rectal cancer following preoperative combined modality therapy. Implications for sphincter preservation. Ann Surg 2007;245:88–93.

65. Branagan G, Chave H, Fuller C, et al. Can magnetic resonance imaging predict circumferential margins and TNM stage in rectal cancer? Dis Colon Rectum 2004;47:1317–22.

66. Burton S, Brown G, Daniels I, et al. MRI identified prognostic features of tumors in distal sigmoid, rectosigmoid, and upper rectum: treatment with radiotherapy and chemotherapy. Int J Radiat Oncol Biol Phys 2006;65:445–51.

67. Rutten H, Sebag-Montefiore D, Glynne-Jones R, et al. Capecitabine, oxaliplatin, radiotherapy, and excision (CORE) in patients with MRI-defined locally advanced rectal adenocarcinoma: results of an international multicenter phase II study. Proc ASCO 2006;24:153s.
68. Baik SH, Kim NK, Lee YC, et al. Prognostic significance of circumferential resection margin following total mesorectal excision and adjuvant chemoradiotherapy in patients with rectal cancer. Ann Surg Oncol 2007;14:462–9.
69. Sebag-Montefiore D, Steele R, Quirke P, et al. Routine short course pre-operative radiotherapy or selective post-op chemoradiotherapy for resectable rectal cancer? Preliminary results of the MRC CR07 randomised trial. Proc ASCO 2006;24:148s.
70. Marijnen CA, Nagtegaal ID, Kapiteijn E, et al. Radiotherapy does not compensate for positive resection margins in rectal cancer patients: report of a multicenter randomized trial. Int J Radiat Oncol Biol Phys 2003;55:1311–20.
71. Habr-Gama A, Santinho B, de Souza PM, et al. Low rectal cancer. Impact of radiation and chemotherapy on surgical treatment. Dis Colon Rectum 1998;41:1087–96.
72. Gavioli M, Bagni A, Piccagli I, et al. Usefulness of endorectal ultrasound after preoperative radiotherapy in rectal cancer. Dis Colon Rectum 2000;43:1075–83.
73. Hiotis SP, Weber SM, Cohen AM, et al. Assessing the predictive value of clinical complete response to neoadjuvant therapy for rectal cancer: an analysis of 488 patients. J Am Coll Surg 2002;194:131–6.
74. Dzik-Jurask A, Domenig C, George M, et al. Diffusion MRI for prediction of response of rectal cancer to chemoradiation. Lancet 2002;360:307–8.
75. Glynne-Jones R, Wallace M, Livingstone JI, et al. Complete clinical response after preoperative chemoradiation in rectal cancer: is a "wait and see" policy justified? Dis Colon Rectum 2008;51:10–20.
76. Borschitz T, Wachtlin D, Mohler M, et al. Neoadjuvant chemoradiation and local excision for T2-3 rectal cancer. Ann Surg Oncol 2008;15:712–20.
77. van Cutsem E, Lang I, D'haens G, et al. KRAS status and efficacy in the first-line treatment of patients with metastatic colorectal cancer (mCRC) treated with FOLFIRI with or without cetuximab: the CRYSTA experience. Proc ASCO 2008;26:1006s.
78. Chung KY, Minsky B, Schrag D, et al. Phase I trial of preoperative cetuximab with concurrent continuous infusion 5-fluorouracil and pelvic radiation in patients with local-regionally advanced rectal cancer. Proc ASCO 2006;24:161s.
79. Stein DE, Mahmoud NN, Anne PR, et al. Longer time interval between completion of neoadjuvant chemoradiation and surgical resection does not improve downstaging of rectal carcinoma. Dis Colon Rectum 2003;46:448–53.
80. Guillem JG, Chessin DB, Cohen AM, et al. Long term oncologic outcome following preoperative combined modality therapy and total mesorectal excision of locally advanced rectal cancer. Ann Surg 2005;241:829–38.
81. Valentini V, Coco C, Picciocchi A, et al. Does downstaging predict improved outcome after preoperative chemoradiation for extraperitoneal locally advanced rectal cancer? A long term analysis of 165 patients. Int J Radiat Oncol Biol Phys 2002;53:664–74.
82. Capirci C, Valentini V, Cionini L, et al. Prognostic value of pathologic complete response after neoadjuvant therapy in locally advanced rectal cancer: long-term analysis of 566 ypCR patients. Int J Radiat Oncol Biol Phys 2008;72:99–107.
83. Bertolini F, Bengala C, Losi L, et al. Prognostic and predictive value of baseline and post treatment molecular marker expression in locally advanced rectal

cancer treated with neoadjuvant chemoradiotherapy. Int J Radiat Oncol Biol Phys 2007;68:1455–61.

84. Johnston PG. Prognostic markers of local relapse in rectal cancer: are we any further forward? J Clin Oncol 2006;24:4049–50.

85. Unsal D, Under A, Akyuerk N, et al. Matrix metalloproteinase-9 expression correlated with tumor response in patients with locally advanced rectal cancer undergoing preoperative chemoradiotherapy. Int J Radiat Oncol Biol Phys 2007;67: 196–203.

86. Kuremsky JG, Tepper JE, McLeod HL. Biomarkers for response to neoadjuvant chemoradiation for rectal cancer. Int J Radiat Oncol Biol Phys 2009;74:673–88.

87. Konski A, Li T, Sigurdson E, et al. Use of molecular imaging to predict clinical outcome in patients with rectal cancer after preoperative chemotherapy and radiation. Int J Radiat Oncol Biol Phys 2009;74:55–9.

88. Aristu JJ, Arbea L, Rodriguez J, et al. Phase I-II trial of concurrent capecitabine and oxaliplatin with preoperative intensity modulated radiotherapy in patients with locally advanced rectal cancer. Int J Radiat Oncol Biol Phys 2008;71:748–55.

89. Meyer J, Czito B, Yin FF, et al. Advanced radiation therapy technologies in the treatment of rectal and anal cancer: intensity-modulated photon therapy and proton therapy. Clin Colorectal Cancer 2007;6:348–56.

90. Tatsuzaki H, Urie MM, Willett CG. 3-D comparative study of proton vs. x-ray radiation therapy for rectal cancer. Int J Radiat Oncol Biol Phys 1991;22(2):369–74.

91. Callister MD, Ezzell GA, Gunderson LL. IMRT reduces the dose to small bowel and other pelvic organs in the preoperative treatment of rectal cancer. Int J Radiat Oncol Biol Phys 2006;66:s290.

92. Myerson RJ, Garofalo MC, El Naqa I, et al. Elective clinical target volumes for conformal therapy in anorectal cancer: a radiation therapy oncology group consensus panel contouring atlas. Int J Radiat Oncol Biol Phys 2009;74:824–30.

93. Roels S, Duthoy W, Haustermans K, et al. Definition and delineation of the clinical target volume for rectal cancer. Int J Radiat Oncol Biol Phys 2006;65:1129–42.

Adjuvant Therapy for Colon Cancer

Leonard B. Saltz, MD[a,b]

KEYWORDS

• Adjuvant therapy • Colorectal cancer • Disease-free survival
• 5-FluorouracilU

Patients are not at risk of dying from tumor that has been removed; they are at risk of dying from residual microscopic disease not removed at the time of operation. Thus, the goal of an adjuvant treatment, be it chemotherapy, radiation therapy, immunotherapy, or dietary and lifestyle manipulations, is to eradicate any residual, albeit microscopic, metastatic disease that might remain. If the surgeon has truly "gotten it all," then the patient is cured and there is no need or justification for subjecting the patient to any further treatment. It is because of the inability to determine definitively who does and who does not harbor micrometastatic disease that adjuvant therapy, predominantly chemotherapy, is administered to large numbers of patients with resected colon cancer, many of whom may have already been rendered disease-free by their operation.

Clinical stage remains the best prognostic indicator of the risk of what is somewhat inaccurately referred to as recurrence. Thus, stage is the best predictor of whether the patient harbors undetected microscopic stage IV disease. Stage is determined by the depth of tumor penetration into or through the bowel wall and the number of lymph nodes involved with cancer. Present recommendations are for the examination of an absolute minimum of at least 12 lymph nodes to assure accurate resection and staging. Adequate nodal examination reflects a combination of adequate nodal resection on the part of the surgeon, plus adequate nodal inspection on the part of the pathologist.

Stage I disease carries an excellent prognosis, and at present there are no compelling data to support adjuvant chemotherapy for patients with this early-stage disease. Stage II colon cancer also has a relatively good prognosis after operation alone and represents the most complicated and contentious area in decisions regarding the use of adjuvant chemotherapy. Stage III colorectal cancer (CRC) (TanyN$_{1-2}$M$_0$) represents a group at a higher risk of recurrence, and this population is routinely given adjuvant chemotherapy in the absence of a medical or psychiatric contraindication.

[a] Colorectal Oncology Section, Department of Medicine, Memorial Sloan Kettering Cancer Center, New York, NY 10065, USA
[b] Department of Medicine, Weill Medical College of Cornell University, New York, NY 10065, USA
E-mail address: saltzl@mskcc.org

Surg Oncol Clin N Am 19 (2010) 819–827
doi:10.1016/j.soc.2010.07.005
1055-3207/10/$ – see front matter © 2010 Elsevier Inc. All rights reserved.

Extensive retrospective data have resulted in the segregation of patients with stage III cancer into 3 subgroups based on T category and N category within stage III (IIIA: T1–2, N1; IIIB: T3–4, N1; IIIC: T0–4, N2).[1] The 5-year observed survival rates for these 3 subcategories were 60%, 42%, and 27%, respectively ($P<.001$), with surgery alone indicating the heterogeneity of stage III cancer and the importance of this subcategorization in anticipating prognosis. Similar differences were calculated after stratification for treatment reporting a 5-year observed survival rate of 71%, 51%, and 33% with surgery plus adjuvant fluoropyrimidine chemotherapy for each subgroup, respectively. The data supporting the use of adjuvant therapy in patients with colon cancer are reviewed in later discussion.

HISTORICAL DEVELOPMENT OF ADJUVANT THERAPY

Initial adjuvant trials in colon cancer were negative, due in large part to their being extremely undersized (as few as 30–50 patients per arm), based on unrealistically high expectations of the effect of chemotherapy. The first adequately powered study to address the question was the US Intergroup Trial INT-0035.[2] In this trial, patients receiving 1 year of 5-fluorouracil (5-FU), plus the putative immunomodulator levamisole, experienced a 33% risk reduction compared with the surgery-only control group. In retrospect, levamisole has been shown to be an inactive agent; however, the trial was the first to give adequate doses of 5-FU to a large enough patient population to discern an effect. Subsequently, INT-0089 demonstrated that 6 months of adjuvant bolus 5-FU/leucovorin (LV) (Mayo Clinic Schedule or Roswell Park Schedule) showed a similar benefit to 1 year of bolus 5-FU/levamisole, with no further added benefit of concurrent addition of levamisole to an LV-containing regimen.[3]

Studies of the oral fluoropyrimidines capecitabine and uracil and ftorafur (UFT) have demonstrated that each of these is an acceptable alternative to parenteral 5-FU/LV in the adjuvant setting. In a study powered to evaluate noninferiority of capecitabine versus the Mayo Clinic bolus 5-FU/LV schedule, noninferiority was demonstrated.[4] Similar results (noninferiority of an oral fluoropyrimidine vs Mayo Clinic 5-FU/LV) were demonstrated in the National Surgical Adjuvant Breast and Bowel Project (NSABP) C-06 Trial for the oral agent UFT plus oral LV, although UFT is not commercially available in the United States.[5,6]

OXALIPLATIN-BASED COMBINATION CHEMOTHERAPY REGIMENS

In the Multicenter International Study of Oxaliplatin/5FU-LV in the Adjuvant Treatment of Colon cancer (MOSAIC) trial, 2246 patients (60% stage III and 40% stage II) were randomly assigned to receive either bolus plus infusional 5-FU/LV on an every-other-week schedule (LV5FU2), or the same schedule plus oxaliplatin, which results in a regimen known as FOLFOX-4.[7] Updated efficacy results have now been reported (**Table 1**).[8] Five-year disease-free survival (DFS) was 73.3% for the FOLFOX group and 67.4% in the 5-FU/LV group (hazard ratio [HR] = 0.80; 95% confidence interval [CI], 0.68–0.93; $P = .003$). The 6-year overall survival (OS) rates were 78.5% for the FOLFOX group and 76.0% in the 5-FU/LV group (HR = 0.84; 95% CI, 0.71–1.00; $P = .046$); corresponding 6-year OS rates for patients with stage III disease were 72.9% and 68.7%, respectively (HR = 0.80; 95% CI, 0.65–0.97; $P = .023$). No improvement in OS was seen with the addition of oxaliplatin in patients with stage II disease.

Toxicities were notable for a 12% incidence of grade 3 sensory neuropathy, which remained at grade 3 in 1% of the patients at 1-year follow-up. Long-term neurotoxicity is a major concern, with 27% of patients having some residual neurotoxicity 1 year after the end of treatment and 11% of patients having some residual neurotoxicity

Table 1 Efficacy outcomes of FOLFOX versus 5-FU/LV (MOSAIC Trial)				
	Stage III 6-y OS	Stage III 5-y DFS	Stage II 6-y OS	Stage II 5-y DFS
FOLFOX	72.9%	66.4%	85.0%	83.7%
5-FU/LV	68.7%	58.9%	83.3%	79.9%
P Value	P = .023	P = .005	P = .65	P = .258

Abbreviations: DFS, disease-free survival; OS, overall survival.
Data from Andre T, Boni C, Navarro M, et al: Improved overall survival with oxaliplatin, fluorouracil, and leucovorin as adjuvant treatment in stage II or III colon cancer in the MOSAIC Trial. J Clin Oncol 2009;27:3109–16.

after 4 years of follow-up. It is reasonable to assume that toxicity, which has not resolved after 4 years, is likely to be permanent.

The NSABP C-07 trial evaluated the addition of oxaliplatin to weekly bolus 5-FU/LV (Roswell Park Schedule), randomly assigning 2407 patients with stage II (29%) or stage III colon cancer to half a year of 5-FU/LV (500 mg/m^2 bolus weekly for 6 of every 8 weeks) with or without oxaliplatin (85 mg/m^2 administered on weeks 1, 3, and 5 of every 8-week cycle). With median 34-month follow-up, 3-year DFS for the oxaliplatin/bolus 5-FU/LV (FLOX) arm was 77% versus 72% for bolus 5-FU/LV, with corresponding 21% risk reduction (HR 0.79). However, toxicity was prominent in both groups, with high incidences of grade 3 and 4 diarrhea. Hospitalization for diarrhea or dehydration was required in 5% of patients receiving oxaliplatin and 3% of the control group.

More recently, the combination of capecitabine plus oxaliplatin (CapeOx) has been compared with 5-FU/LV in the NO16968 trial.[9] This trial, thus far reported only in abstract form, shows a statistically significant improvement in 3-year DFS (the prespecified primary end point of the trial) for the patients on the CapeOx arm. This result would seem to justify use of CapeOx as an alternative to FOLFOX or FLOX. It should be noted that CapeOx requires a highly reliable, motivated patient to assure adequate and accurate compliance with the medication schedule. Because patients require intravenous administration of oxaliplatin in the CapeOx regimen, it remains a matter of individual subjective judgment as to whether the fully parenteral or parenteral plus oral regimen is more convenient for the patient.

Given the results of the MOSAIC, C-07, and NO16968 trials, oxaliplatin plus a fluoropyrimidine should be regarded as standard adjuvant treatment for completely resected stage III colon cancer and should be regarded as an appropriate consideration for high-risk patients with stage II cancer. Head-to-head comparisons of the FOLFOX and FLOX regimens are not, and will never be, available. However, based on the apparent superior toxicity profile, the FOLFOX regimen is generally preferred. The unreported AVANT trial provides randomized comparison of a FOLFOX and CapeOx-based regimen.

NEGATIVE TRIALS: IRINOTECAN, BEVACIZUMAB, AND CETUXIMAB

A classic paradigm of drug development has been to establish in the metastatic setting that a combination of a standard treatment plus a new agent is superior to that standard treatment alone. Having established efficacy in the metastatic setting, investigators then move that new regimen into the adjuvant setting to attempt to increase the cure rate. However, all too often practitioners make the premature decision to adopt such new combinations into their standard adjuvant practice before the adjuvant trials have been completed. As demonstrated by the results of irinotecan, bevacizumab, and cetuximab, all of which are part of the standard management of metastatic disease, such premature conclusions are unwarranted and may place patients at risk of needless and potentially dangerous toxicity.

Irinotecan

Following the demonstration that irinotecan conferred a survival advantage in the metastatic setting, the Cancer and Leukemia Group B Intergroup trial, C89803, evaluated the IFL weekly irinotecan/5-FU/LV bolus schedule compared with the bolus Roswell Park 5-FU/LV schedule in patients with stage III CRC.[10] The addition of irinotecan to bolus 5-FU/LV demonstrated no clinical benefit in either DFS or OS, and a significantly higher early death rate was observed in patients randomized to the IFL arm as well as significant increases in grade 3 or 4 neutropenia and febrile neutropenia.

Similarly disappointing results were seen with the FOLFIRI (biweekly irinotecan plus 48-hour infusional 5-FU) regimen. The Action to Control Cardiovascular Risk in Diabetes (ACCORD) II trial randomized 400 patients with high-risk stage III disease (4 or more nodes positive or obstructed or perforated colon cancers) to biweekly infusional 5-FU/LV with or without irinotecan.[11] With a median follow-up of 36 months, event-free survival was not significantly different between the arms but trended toward inferiority of the irinotecan-containing arm. There were significant imbalances in several important prognostic factors between the arms that favored the control arm; however, even in models adjusting for these imbalances, the irinotecan-containing arm remained nonsignificantly inferior. In a subset analysis of the MOSAIC trial involving FOLFOX, a similar group of high-risk patients with stage III cancer (4 or more positive nodes) actually achieved the most benefit from the addition of oxaliplatin, suggesting that this high-risk group would offer the greatest chance for irinotecan to show a favorable result; yet this irinotecan trial was clearly negative.

The Pan European Trial of Advanced Colon Cancer (PETACC)-3 trial compared biweekly infusional 5-FU/LV to the same regimen plus 180 mg of irinotecan (the FOLFIRI regimen) in 3278 patients, 2333 of who had stage III colon cancer and made up the group that was evaluated for the primary efficacy analysis.[12] There was no significant difference in the prespecified primary end point of the trial, which was 3-year DFS in stage III patients (3-year DFS 63% vs 60%, HR 0.89, $P = .107$). A retrospective evaluation of patients with stage III cancer demonstrated a higher percentage of T4 patients in the irinotecan arm compared with the infusional 5-FU/LV alone arm (n = 180 vs 130 patients, 17% vs 13%). However, it should be noted that T category was not included as a potential prognostic variable for modeling in the protocol; thus its inclusion in the modeling is a post hoc analysis. In this risk-adjusted statistical analysis of the stage III data involving T and N category stratification, a significant DFS (HR 0.85, CI 0.74–0.98, $P = .021$) and relapse-free survival (HR 0.82, CI 0.71–0.95, $P = .009$) was identified. Nonetheless, this trial failed to meet its prespecified statistical primary end point of improvement of DFS. Furthermore, the PETAC-3 trial cannot be interpreted in a vacuum; although aspects of this trial suggest some possibility of modest benefit, the ACCORD II and C89803 trials are strongly negative. Based on the aggregate of these 3 large randomized adjuvant trials, irinotecan-containing chemotherapy appears to be clinically ineffective and should not be used in standard practice in the adjuvant setting.

Bevacizumab

A pivotal placebo-controlled phase III trial of IFL versus IFL plus bevacizumab given at 5 mg/kg every 14 days demonstrated a 4.7-month survival benefit to the group receiving bevacizumab. Rare but serious events, such as gastrointestinal perforation and arterial thrombotic events as well as more common but less serious events such as proteinuria and hypertension, were statistically significantly increased in the group receiving bevacizumab. The NSABP, building on the positive adjuvant trials with oxaliplatin and making the assumption that the benefits of adding bevacizumab to IFL would necessarily translate to oxaliplatin-based therapy as well, conducted a 2700-patient randomized trial of FOLFOX versus FOLFOX plus bevacizumab. After the start of this trial, a 1400-patient randomized trial of oxaliplatin-based first-line therapy for metastatic disease plus or minus bevacizumab,[13] although showing a modest, albeit statistically significant 1.4-month improvement in progression-free survival, failed to show either a statistically or clinically significant survival benefit, and the trial showed absolutely no response benefit, raising concerns about the utility of bevacizumab in the adjuvant setting. In a maneuver that is difficult to justify, the NSABP chose to lengthen the duration of bevacizumab to 1 full year. Thus, the trial was 6 months of FOLFOX versus 6 months of FOLFOX plus bevacizumab followed by an additional 6 months of bevacizumab alone.

Had this trial produced a positive result it would, in all likelihood, have been impossible to ever conduct a trial to determine if the additional 6 months of bevacizumab contributed to the outcome. However, that problem did not arise because this trial, reported thus far in abstract form, is negative, having failed to meet its prespecified primary end point of improved 3-year DFS.[14] There was an interesting, albeit clinically irrelevant improvement in DFS at 1 year, suggesting that the indefinite continuation of bevacizumab might improve cancer-specific outcome; however, the toxicity and expense of such prolonged bevacizumab exposure make evaluation or use of such an approach unreasonable. At this time, there is no role for the use of bevacizumab in the adjuvant setting of colon cancer.

Cetuximab

Clinical trials with cetuximab had demonstrated antitumor responses when given both as a single agent and in conjunction with chemotherapy. The North Central Cancer Treatment Group (NCCTG) initiated a phase 3 trial of FOLFOX plus or minus cetuximab in patients with stage III colon cancer. After the start of the trial, only tumors that harbored mutations in the Kirsten rat sarcoma (KRAS) gene were potentially sensitive to cetuximab, and the trial was restructured to further enroll only those patients whose tumors had these mutations. In the autumn of 2009, the Data Safety Monitoring Committee of the NCCTG informed investigators that the trial was being immediately halted because of its futility. A presentation of the data in abstract form revealed no benefit in 3-year DFS or OS with the addition of cetuximab, even to patients with tumors that do not have KRAS mutations.[15] The data from a European trial, PETACC-8, are still maturing; however, at this time it is not appropriate to use cetuximab in the adjuvant setting.

STAGE II COLON CANCER

The utility of adjuvant chemotherapy for patients with stage II colon cancer remains controversial. Stage II CRC (T3–4N0M0) makes up approximately a quarter of newly diagnosed CRC patients and has a good prognosis, with a 72% to 85% OS. However, for high-risk patients with stage II cancer, with either clinical obstruction, perforation, poorly differentiated histology, lymphovascular invasion, or inadequate lymph node sampling (<10 nodes), a generally poorer prognosis can be expected, with an approximate 5-year DFS estimate of 60% to 70%. Although there are no definitive data showing treatment benefit in this group, most data suggest, and most clinicians believe, that such patients are appropriate for treatment along the lines of patients with stage III cancer. Microsatellite instability (MSI) and absence of loss of heterozygosity (LOH) of 18q have been suggested to be favorable prognostic markers, possibly avoiding adjuvant therapy, and are discussed under the heading of molecular markers in later discussion.

A subset analysis of 318 patients with stage II cancer in US Intergroup 0035, randomized to receive either 5-FU and levamisole or surgery alone, demonstrated no difference in 7-year survival rates, 72% for both groups (P = .83).[16]

The quick and simple and reliable (QUASAR) adjuvant trial from the United Kingdom, involving 3289 predominately (91%) patients with stage II CRC with "uncertain indications for adjuvant treatment," 71% of whom had colon as opposed to rectal cancer, demonstrated a modest but statistically significant reduction in recurrence rate (22.2% vs 26.2%; HR 0.78, 95% CI, 0.67–0.91) and an improvement in 5-year survival rate (80.3% vs 77.4%; HR 0.83, 95% CI, 0.71–0.97) with adjuvant chemotherapy compared with observation.[17] In the IMPACT (International Multicenter Pooled Analysis of Colon Cancer Trial) study, a pooled analysis of 5 European trials involving 1016 patients with stage II colon cancer randomized to adjuvant 5-FU/LV versus observation showed a 5-year survival of 82% versus 80%, respectively.[18] This analysis trended strongly toward, but did not reach, statistical significance.

The Surveillance, Epidemiology, and End-Results Medicare Analysis identified 3151 patients with stage II cancer, with no high-risk features using the Medicare database.[19] Approximately 27% of these elderly Medicare patients received adjuvant chemotherapy (predominately 5-FU/LV). With an OS rate of 78% for chemotherapy patients versus 75% for observed patients, this nonrandomized analysis suggests minimal benefit of adjuvant chemotherapy for patients with stage II CRC.

Multiple meta-analyses have attempted to determine the benefit of chemotherapy in patients with stage II CRC: the pooled Intergroup Meta-analysis evaluated 3302 stage II and III patients with colon cancer from 7 randomized trials comparing adjuvant 5-FU/LV or 5-FU/levamisole versus observation.[20] Patients with stage II colon cancer did not demonstrate a survival advantage (81% vs 80%, P = .113) in this analysis.

The Cancer Care Ontario Practice Guideline Initiative Gastrointestinal Cancer Disease Site Group systematically reviewed 37 trials and 11 meta-analyses published after 1987.[21] A separate meta-analysis sanctioned by American Society of Clinical Oncology was performed on a subset of 12 trials (4187 patients) with an observation arm and at least one 5-FU–based adjuvant chemotherapy arm for patients with stage II colon cancer.[22] The mortality risk ratio for patients with stage II CRC did not reach statistical significance (HR 0.87, 95% CI, 0.75–1.10, P = .07).

A subset analysis of the MOSAIC Trial demonstrated no statistically significant advantage of the addition of oxaliplatin to LV5FU2 in patients with stage II cancer; however, this subset was too small to adequately address this question.[7] However, in the 12% (108 of 899) of patients with stage II cancer with high-risk features (T4 primary, perforation, obstruction, or vascular invasion), a strong trend toward improved outcome with the addition of oxaliplatin was seen.

MOLECULAR MARKERS

At present, there are no validated markers to assist in the selection of either patients who do or do not need chemotherapy, or specific chemotherapy agents, for an individual patient in the adjuvant setting. The Eastern Cooperative Oncology Group E5202 trial is evaluating the role of chemotherapy in higher-risk patients with stage II CRC as defined by the absence of high MSI and intact 18q status. Patients with microsatellite stable disease and/or LOH at chromosome 18q are assigned to treatment with modified FOLFOX-6 and randomized to receive bevacizumab or not, whereas patients with high MSI and no 18q LOH are assigned to the observation alone arm. Accrual is continuing.

Some studies have suggested that tumors with high MSI (either by direct measurement or by demonstration of deficient mismatch repair protein [MMR] on immunohistochemical staining) do not benefit, or may even suffer a detriment, from 5-FU/LV. An analysis of MSI from archival tissues from 4 NSABP adjuvant chemotherapy trials demonstrated no prognostic correlation and no trend toward a correlation between high MSI and OS ($P = .67$).[23] However, more recently, Sargent and colleagues[24] reported on 457 stage II or III patients with colon cancer, with tumor samples available, who were randomized to 5-FU–based chemotherapy versus observation in National Cancer Institute cooperative group trials (**Table 2**). Fifteen percent of these patients were found to have tumors that were MMR deficient. In patients with these MMR-deficient tumors, no benefit from 5-FU was seen in DFS. In patients with stage II cancer, with MMR-deficient tumors, treatment with 5-FU was associated with decreased OS. These data support the use of MMR evaluation in patients with stage II cancer and indicate that single-agent fluoropyrimidine should not be used in patients with MMR-deficient tumors. Because oxaliplatin was not available and therefore not used in the patients studied, these data do not comment on the role of MMR in the effectiveness of FOLFOX or other oxaliplatin-containing regimens.

Pharmacogenomic studies are attempting to identify those patients who may be at higher risk of toxicity from specific agents. These studies may identify subgroups for whom one therapy or another is more effective or safer, or both. However, this remains an investigational approach at this time.

SUMMARY AND CLINICAL RECOMMENDATIONS

The FOLFOX regimen is the current regimen of choice for patients with stage III cancer and for at least high-risk patients with stage II cancer. Although the FOLFOX-4 regimen was involved in the registration trial, the modified FOLFOX-6 regimen, with a simplified 5-FU/LV dosing schedule compared with FOLFOX-, is what is most widely used in practice. Modified FOLFOX-6 has served as the basis for the most recent US Cooperative Group studies involving the FOLFOX regimen. The CapeOx and FLOX

Table 2			
Mismatch repair status as a predictor of benefit from 5-FU			
MMR Status	**Treatment Arm**	**5-y DFS (%)**	**P value**
MMR-deficient	Observation	76	P = .56
N = 70	5-FU	72	
MMR-proficient	Observation	53	P = .02
N = 387	5-FU	64	

Data from Sargent DJ, Marsoni S, Monges G, et al: Defective mismatch repair as a predictive marker for lack of efficacy of fluorouracil-based adjuvant therapy in colon cancer. J Clin Oncol 2010;28:3219–26.

regimens are acceptable alternatives. Trials of irinotecan, bevacizumab, and cetuximab have been negative in the adjuvant setting. Therefore, these agents should not be used for this purpose. In those patients who are not considered appropriate for oxaliplatin-based therapy, either 5-FU/LV, or the oral fluoropyrimidines capecitabine or UFT plus leucovorin would seem to be reasonable options.

Adjuvant chemotherapy for stage II colon cancer remains a topic of some controversy. Virtually all patients with stage II cancer deserve a medical oncology consultation for a frank discussion of the potential benefits, including a realistic assessment of the relatively small, but potentially real, incremental benefits of treatment. The decision to give adjuvant chemotherapy to low-risk patients with stage II colon cancer should be an informed decision comparing a possible OS advantage of at most 2% to 4% and a 0.5% to 1% risk of mortality with chemotherapy, in addition to chemotherapy-related morbidities. The available clinical trials and meta-analyses do not clearly settle the issue for or against adjuvant chemotherapy for low-risk patients with stage II colon cancer; however, evidence suggests that patients with tumors showing deficient MMR proteins should not be treated with single-agent fluoropyrimidines.

No molecular markers have been shown to be clearly of benefit in selecting patients for adjuvant therapy at this time, as attempts to develop a gene signature to identify those patients who do or do not need treatment have thus far been unsuccessful. At present, there is no utility to molecular analysis (other than MMR as mentioned earlier) in the management of patients with stage II and III cancer.

REFERENCES

1. Greene F, Stewart A, Norton H. A new TNM staging strategy for node-positive (stage III) colon cancer: an analysis of 50,042 patients. Ann Surg 2002;236: 416–21.
2. Moertel C, Fleming T, Macdonald J, et al. Levamisole and fluorouracil for adjuvant therapy of resected colon carcinoma. N Engl J Med 1990;322:352.
3. Haller DG, Catalano PJ, Macdonald JS, et al. Phase III study of fluorouracil, leucovorin, and levamisole in high-risk stage II and III colon cancer: final report of Intergroup 0089. J Clin Oncol 2005;23:8671–8.
4. Van Cutsem E, Twelves C, Cassidy J, et al. Oral capecitabine compared with intravenous fluorouracil plus leucovorin in patients with metastatic colorectal cancer: results of a large phase III study. J Clin Oncol 2001;19:4097–106.
5. Saltz LB, Leichman CG, Young CW, et al. A fixed-ratio combination of uracil and ftorafur (UFT) with low dose leucovorin. An active oral regimen for advanced colorectal cancer. Cancer 1995;75:782–5.
6. Lembersky BC, Wieand HS, Petrelli NJ, et al. Oral uracil and tegafur plus leucovorin compared with intravenous fluorouracil and leucovorin in stage II and III carcinoma of the colon: results from National Surgical Adjuvant Breast and Bowel Project Protocol C-06. J Clin Oncol 2006;24:2059–64.
7. Andre T, Boni C, Mounedji-Boudiaf L, et al. Oxaliplatin, fluorouracil, and leucovorin as adjuvant treatment for colon cancer. N Engl J Med 2004;350:2343–51.
8. Andre T, Boni C, Navarro M, et al. Improved overall survival with oxaliplatin, fluorouracil, and leucovorin as adjuvant treatment in stage II or III colon cancer in the MOSAIC trial. J Clin Oncol 2009;27:3109–16.
9. Haller D, Tabernero J, Maroun J, et al. 5LBA First efficacy findings from a randomized phase III trial of capecitabine + oxaliplatin vs. bolus 5-FU/LV for stage III colon cancer (NO16968/XELOXA study). Proceedings of European Society of Medical Oncology (ESMO) 2009;7:4.

10. Saltz LB, Neidzweicki D, Hollis D, et al. Irinotecan fluorouracil plus leucovorin is not superior to fluorouracil plus leucovorin alone as adjuvant treatment for stage III colon cancer: results of CALGB 89803. J Clin Oncol 2007;25:3456–61.
11. Ychou M, Raoul J, Douillard JY, et al. A phase III randomised trial of LV5FU2 + irinotecan versus LV5FU2 alone in adjuvant high-risk colon cancer (FNCLCC Accord02/FFCD9802). Ann Oncol 2009;20:674–80.
12. Van Cutsem E, Labianca R, Hossfeld G, et al. Randomized phase III trial comparing biweekly infusional fluorouracil/leucovorin alone or with irinotecan in the adjuvant treatment of stage III colon cancer: PETACC-3. J Clin Oncol 2009; 27:3117–25.
13. Saltz LB, Clarke S, Diaz-Rubio E, et al. Bevacizumab in combination with oxaliplatin-based chemotherapy as first-line therapy in metastatic colorectal cancer: a randomized phase III study. J Clin Oncol 2008;26:2013–9.
14. Wolmark N, Yothers G, O'Connell MJ, et al. A phase III trial comparing mFOL-FOX6 to mFOLFOX6 plus bevacizumab in stage II or III carcinoma of the colon: results of NSABP protocol C-08 [abstract]. J Clin Oncol 2009;27(Suppl):LBA4.
15. Alberts SR, Sargent DJ, Smyrk CJ, et al. Adjuvant mFOLFOX6 with or without cetuximab (Cmab) in KRAS wild-type (WT) patients (pts) with resected stage III colon cancer (CC): results from NCCTG intergroup phase III trial N0147 [abstract]. J Clin Oncol 2010;28(Suppl):CRA3507.
16. Moertel CG, Fleming TR, Macdonald JS, et al. Intergroup study of fluorouracil plus levamisole as adjuvant therapy for stage II/Duke's B2 colon cancer. J Clin Oncol 1995;13:2936–43.
17. QUASAR Collaborative Group. Adjuvant chemotherapy versus observation in patients with colorectal cancer: a randomised study. Lancet 2007;370:2020–9.
18. Aarnio M, Sankila R, Pukkala E, et al. Cancer risk in mutation carriers of DNA-mismatch-repair genes. Int J Cancer 1999;81:214–8.
19. Schrag D, Rifas-Shiman S, Saltz L, et al. Adjuvant chemotherapy use for Medicare beneficiaries with stage II colon cancer. J Clin Oncol 2002;20:3999–4005.
20. Gill S, Loprinzi CL, Sargent DJ, et al. Pooled analysis of fluorouracil-based adjuvant therapy for stage II and III colon cancer: who benefits and by how much? J Clin Oncol 2004;22:1797–806.
21. Figueredo A, Charette ML, Maroun J, et al. Adjuvant therapy for stage II colon cancer: a systematic review from the cancer care Ontario program in evidence-based care's gastrointestinal cancer disease site group. J Clin Oncol 2004;22:3395–407.
22. Benson AB 3rd, Schrag D, Somerfield MR, et al. American Society of Clinical Oncology recommendations on adjuvant chemotherapy for stage II colon cancer. J Clin Oncol 2004;22:3408–19.
23. Kim GP, Colangelo LH, Wieand HS, et al. Prognostic and predictive roles of high-degree microsatellite instability in colon cancer: a national cancer institute-national surgical adjuvant breast and bowel project collaborative study. J Clin Oncol 2007;25:767–72.
24. Sargent DJ, Marsoni S, Monges G, et al. Defective mismatch repair as a predictive marker for lack of efficacy of fluorouracil-based adjuvant therapy in colon cancer. J Clin Oncol 2010;28:3219–26.

Complete Clinical Response after Neoadjuvant Chemoradiation for Distal Rectal Cancer

Angelita Habr-Gama, MD, PhD[a,b,]*, Rodrigo Perez, MD, PhD[b,c],
Igor Proscurshim, MD[b,d], Joaquim Gama-Rodrigues, MD, PhD[a,b]

KEYWORDS

- Clinical response • Neoadjuvant chemoradiation
- Distal rectal cancer • Multimodal treatment

Multimodality treatment of rectal cancer, with the combination of radiation therapy, chemotherapy, and surgery has become the preferred approach to locally advanced rectal cancer.[1–4] The considerably high local recurrence rates observed after radical surgery alone has led to the use and recommendation for additional therapy either before or after surgery for T3/T4 or N+ tumors.[5] In this setting, to avoid overtreatment of patients with early-stage disease, preoperative treatment with radiation therapy with or without concomitant chemotherapy requires optimal radiological staging because there is no pathologic confirmation of exact TNM parameters. However, there is a theoretic benefit of exposing unscarred tissue with optimal oxygen delivery to both radiation and chemotherapy as opposed to postoperative treatment. The results from randomized controlled trials suggest that the neoadjuvant approach seems to be superior for local disease control, even in the setting of appropriate surgical technique (total mesorectal excision).[1] The use of neoadjuvant chemoradiation therapy (CRT) has resulted in additional benefits such as reduced toxicity rates, significant tumor downsizing and downstaging, better chance of sphincter preservation, and improved functional results (compared with postoperative CRT).[1,6] In a multicenter study of patients undergoing

[a] University of Sao Paulo, Av Dr Enéas de Carvalho Aguiar 255, Sao Paulo, SP 05403-000, Brazil
[b] Angelita & Joaquim Gama Institute, Rua Manoel da Nobrega 1564, Ibirapuera, Sao Paulo, SP 04001-005, Brazil
[c] Colorectal Surgery Division, Department of Gastroenterology, University of Sao Paulo, Sao Paulo, Brazil
[d] General Surgery Department, University of Sao Paulo, Sao Paulo, Brazil
* Corresponding author. Angelita & Joaquim Gama Institute, Rua Manoel da Nobrega 1564, Ibirapuera, Sao Paulo, SP 04001-005, Brazil.
E-mail address: gamange@uol.com.br

Surg Oncol Clin N Am 19 (2010) 829–845
doi:10.1016/j.soc.2010.08.001
1055-3207/10/$ – see front matter © 2010 Elsevier Inc. All rights reserved.

neoadjuvant CRT for clinically stage II disease (staged by either endorectal ultrasound or magnetic resonance imaging), more than 20% of the patients staged as N0 were found to harbor lymph node metastases in their tumors on pathologic examination. Considering that these patients underwent neoadjuvant CRT, even greater rates of nodal disease underestimation might be expected. The investigators concluded that radiological inaccuracy (particularly for nodal disease) may justify, and possibly warrant, overtreatment of patients with rectal cancer by the use of neoadjuvant CRT.[7] There is a subset of patients with early-stage disease (particularly T2N0) who may also benefit from neoadjuvant CRT despite there having been no demonstration of improved local disease control in randomized trials. Patients with distal T2N0 rectal cancers are at higher risk for developing local disease recurrence compared with the mid- and upper rectal locations.[8] In addition to the potential benefits in terms of local disease control in this high-risk group of patients, neoadjuvant CRT could also improve the chance for sphincter preservation in these patients, allowing for ultralow or even intersphincteric resections.[9]

RATIONALE FOR THE INVESTIGATION OF A NONOPERATIVE APPROACH

Radical surgery with total mesorectal excision remains the mainstay of treatment of distal rectal cancer and is considered by many to be necessary regardless of tumor response to neoadjuvant CRT. However, it has been associated with high rates of immediate morbidity and mortality. For immediate morbidity, an anastomotic leak is one of the most important complications and may occur in up to 12% of cases.[1,10] Overall, perioperative mortality may reach 2% to 3% in patients managed by radical surgery. Perioperative mortality is significantly higher, reaching up to 13% of patients with anastomotic leaks, when temporary diversion is not performed.[11,12] The requirement for a temporary stoma may add additional morbidity related to stoma closure and should be considered in the cumulative morbidity of rectal cancer management.[13] Preoperative radiation may lead to a significant increase in the risk of leaks; however, prospective randomized trials have failed to demonstrate the differences described in previous retrospective analysis.[1,11,12]

Tumor regression after neoadjuvant CRT may be observed not only in the primary tumor (within the rectal wall) but also in perirectal metastatic lymph nodes. This finding has been supported by the observation of a shift toward earlier disease staging in patients treated preoperatively with CRT, for whom the rates of stage II or III disease are markedly decreased compared with patients managed by surgery and postoperative CRT.[1,6]

Tumor regression after neoadjuvant CRT may be complete, leading to an absence of residual neoplasia in the resected specimen, known as complete pathologic response or ypT0N0M0 (ypCR).[14]

Therefore, the rationale for a nonoperative approach to patients with rectal cancer is to avoid a significantly morbid procedure in patients with complete tumor regression after neoadjuvant CRT.

FACTORS INFLUENCING TUMOR REGRESSION

In a review of phase II and phase III studies including variable regimens of neoadjuvant CRT, several factors were found to be associated with higher rates of ypCR after radical surgery. The use of fluorouracil (5-FU) by continuous venous infusion, the delivery of a radiation therapy dose higher than 45 Gy, and the use of an additional drug combine with 5-FU have all been associated with increased rates of ypCR.[15]

Another factor that has frequently been associated with complete tumor regression is the interval between CRT completion and surgery. Radical surgery has traditionally been recommended to be performed 6 weeks after CRT completion.[1,10] In the authors' experience with neoadjuvant CRT, initial assessment of tumor response should be performed no less than 8 weeks after CRT completion.[16,17] No strong evidence exists to guide optimal timing for response assessment for rectal cancer; however, retrospective data indicate that longer periods after CRT completion may be associated with higher rates of tumor downstaging. Several retrospective studies have shown that patients managed by radical surgery 7 to 8 weeks after CRT completion had increased rates of ypCR.[18–20] In one of the studies, patients managed by surgery 7 weeks after CRT had improved outcomes.[18] In a recent retrospective review of patients managed by neoadjuvant CRT in a single institution, there was a steep increase in ypCR rates when surgery was performed 7 weeks after CRT completion. These ypCR rates stabilized after 12 weeks from CRT completion.[20]

An argument for performing surgery shortly (<8 weeks) after CRT completion is the risk of leaving the tumor in situ for prolonged periods of time, with potential metastatic dissemination of tumor cells during this period. Tumor cell death seems to be related to a process induced by ionizing radiation. It is thought that after exposure to a dose of 44 Gy, the metastatic potential of these tumors is significantly compromised because of the potential decrease in the overall number of surviving cells in the tumor.[21] One recent study analyzed the interval between CRT and surgery and found that a prolonged interval (>8 weeks) between CRT and surgery may not have any associated oncologic compromise. In addition, these patients were associated with less postoperative morbidity, further supporting the safety of assessing tumor response at prolonged intervals.[22]

ASSESSMENT OF TUMOR RESPONSE

Assessment of tumor response may be challenging for even the most experienced colorectal surgeon. Even though clinical symptoms subside in patients with complete clinical response, the specificity of symptoms is low because a significant proportion of patients experience some degree of tumor regression and symptom relief. However, residual disease may still be clinically obvious. Clinical assessment using digital rectal examination and rigid proctoscopy is the mainstay of response assessment. Until now, we have considered clinical assessment to be the major determinant for individualization of treatment strategies such as radical surgery, transanal local excision (particularly with the use of transanal endoscopic microsurgery), or even a nonoperative approach.

Complete clinical response is the absence of residual disease after neoadjuvant CRT. If there is any visible or palpable irregularity or nodule, even after near-complete tumor regression, full-thickness transanal local excision or transanal endoscopic microsurgery should be attempted as a diagnostic procedure. Besides proper surgical technique, full pathologic examination is of paramount importance, because diagnosis of microscopic residual disease may be a challenge for the pathologist. Such procedures should be performed by an experienced pathologist belonging to the multidisciplinary team involved in rectal cancer management. With the incorporation of the transanal endoscopic microsurgery technique, improved lateral and radial margin visualization during local excision may provide excellent specimens which will allow the pathologist to precisely determine margins, tumor regression grade, and other standard pathologic features (**Fig. 1**). Forceps biopsies should not be routinely attempted in these patients, particularly in deciding between complete and incomplete response to neoadjuvant CRT, because the tissue specimens from this procedure are usually small and superficial, leading to an increased risk of false-negative results.

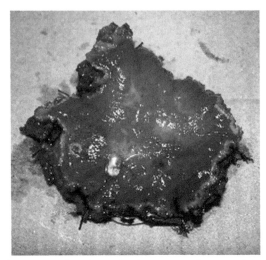

Fig. 1. Specimen after transanal endoscopic microsurgery for a suspicious area after neoadjuvant CRT. Pathology showed a residual ypT1 with significant tumor regression and abundant fibrosis (Mandard TRG2).

In our experience, a subtle whitening of the mucosa and the presence of telangiectasia may be detectable by proctoscopy in some patients with complete clinical regression, and these patients should be considered for an initial nonoperative approach (**Fig. 2**).

Because clinical assessments by rigid proctoscopy and digital rectal examination are two of the most important tools in assessing tumor response to CRT, tumors located higher in the rectum may provide insufficient information for the alternative of a nonoperative approach. In addition, tumors that are not accessible to the surgeon's finger may allow safe anterior resections with less risk for sphincter resection and local recurrence.

Studies performed on the accuracy of clinical assessment of patients with rectal cancer after neoadjuvant CRT showed disappointing sensitivity and specificity. However, these studies used 6-week intervals between CRT completion and response assessment, and therefore could have detected residual disease in patients with

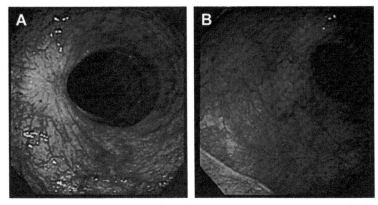

Fig. 2. Endoscopic view of a complete clinical response after neoadjuvant CRT (A). The same study including the dentate line in field of view from proctoscopy (B).

ongoing tumor regression. In addition, the inclusion of different examiners could have biased results, depending on an individual's experience and perception of complete clinical responses.[23]

Carcinoembryonic antigen (CEA) has been extensively used in colorectal cancer management for different purposes. One study of patients undergoing radical surgery alone for rectal cancer found that a decrease in CEA 7 days after rectal resection was associated with improved outcomes, suggesting that initial CEA levels were probably exclusively determined by the primary tumor instead of microscopic undetected metastatic disease.[24] In addition to clinical and radiological assessment of tumor response, determination of CEA levels before and after CRT may also be useful. In a study of more than 500 patients with rectal cancer managed by neoadjuvant CRT, low CEA before treatment was a predictor of ypCR after radical surgery in univariate analysis.[25] Similar findings have been reported in a retrospective analysis of patients undergoing variable neoadjuvant CRT regimens for very low (<2.5 ng/dL) pretreatment CEA levels.[26] In our experience, the decrease or difference between pre-CRT and post-CRT CEA levels were not good predictors of complete tumor regression. Instead, patients with low post-CRT CEA levels, irrespective of pre-CRT CEA levels, had higher rates of complete clinical response and improved outcomes after neoadjuvant therapy.[27]

Radiological assessment of tumor response has been the ultimate challenge in rectal cancer management. Staging of primary tumor depth of penetration and distance from the circumferential margin seem to be adequately provided by endorectal ultrasound and magnetic resonance imaging (metanalyses Santoro). However, in neoadjuvant CRT, distinguishing between residual cancer and transmural fibrosis may be significantly compromised by both ultrasonography and magnetic resonance imaging because these tools rely heavily on morphologic features.[28–30] However, in neoadjuvant CRT, distinguishing between residual cancer and transmural fibrosis may be significantly compromised by both ultrasonography and magnetic resonance imaging because these tools rely heavily on morphologic features.[31,32] Improvements in resolution with these pelvic imaging modalities may provide increased reliability of results in the near future.

The incorporation of positron emission tomography (PET) imaging into the staging work-up provided significant additional information by overlaying metabolic activity data with standard morphology. In addition, PET imaging may also provide an objective estimate of the metabolic activity of a specific area as represented by the standard uptake value measured at various phases of the study. One study of 25 patients with rectal cancer compared the results of baseline PET-computed tomography (CT) before CRT with a second PET-CT performed 6 weeks after CRT completion. All patients included in the study experienced a decrease in maximum standard uptake values (SUV_{max}) between baseline and 6-week PET-CT scans. Also, the final SUV_{max} obtained at 6 weeks was significantly associated with primary tumor downstaging; patients with tumor downstaging exhibited significantly lower SUV_{max} (1.9 vs 3.3; $P = .03$).[33] Even though SUV_{max} obtained at 6 weeks from CRT was associated with tumor downstaging, SUV_{max} did not correlate with final outcome. In another study of 15 patients undergoing baseline PET (before CRT) followed by a second PET 6 weeks after CRT completion, the visual response score was shown to provide superior prediction of tumor downstaging in addition of the extent of pathologic response to CRT.[34] This same group of patients was prospectively followed and outcome analysis showed that patients who developed recurrent disease had significantly lower percentual decrease between baseline and 6-week PET SUV_{max} values. A cutoff of a 62.5% decrease/difference between baseline and 6-week PET SUV_{max} values was a significant predictor of disease-free survival.[35] The same investigators also studied the possibility of tumor response prediction by early sequential PET imaging. In a study of 25 patients undergoing baseline PET, followed by early (10 days after initiation of CRT) PET, the visual response score was able to predict patients who would develop ypCR after CRT. The visual response score could be useful in tailoring treatment of these patients.[36]

These studies each included only a small number of patients, and none of them considered how increased interval periods between CRT and tumor response assessment may influence results. A more recent study examined 30 patients with rectal cancer less than 5 mm from the circumferential margin, as determined by magnetic resonance imaging. All patients underwent CRT, including 65.6 Gy of radiation, and baseline PET-CT and PET-CT performed 8 weeks after CRT were compared. This study found a poor correlation between PET-CT results and final pathologic findings. The sensitivity and specificity for ypCR were 75% and 40%, respectively. Twelve out of 30 patients had a false-negative PET-CT result.[37]

In an earlier study, we performed PET-CT studies in patients with complete clinical response and who were being managed nonoperatively after a variable interval of follow-up. In all 22 patients studied, PET-CT showed no signs of residual disease in the primary site, consistent with the findings of clinical, endoscopic, and radiological assessment. Eight patients with known residual disease after CRT completion also underwent PET-CT and served as a positive control group and all 8 patients were positive by PET-CT for residual disease within the rectal wall. This study suggests that PET-CT may be useful in late assessment of tumor response after nonoperative management of patients with complete clinical response after CRT. It also provides evidence of adequate long-term local and systemic control in patients with complete clinical response.[38] There is an ongoing study at our institution, dedicated to the study of PET-CT in assessing tumor response after neoadjuvant CRT. In this study, all patients undergo a baseline, 6-week post-CRT, and a 12-week post-CRT PET-CT. In addition, patients with sustained complete clinical response and who are not operated on will undergo further PET imaging annually as part of follow-up. The results of this study are not available yet but should provide information on the role of PET-CT imaging in assessing tumor response, and on the benefits of a prolonged (12 weeks vs 6 weeks) interval of assessment in tumor metabolism and downstaging (**Figs. 3** and **4**).

Evaluation of Lymph Node Metastases

The importance of inclusion of the mesorectum within the radiation field of patients undergoing neoadjuvant CRT for rectal cancer is well established.[39] Therefore, this kind of therapy might be expected to have some effect on perirectal nodes, similar to what is observed in the primary tumor. Ultimately, downstaging of rectal cancer may not only be observed in T status but also in N status.

Radiation may have an effect on the overall number of pelvic and perirectal lymph nodes of patients undergoing neoadjuvant radiation therapy followed by radical surgery. Data obtained from the Surveillance, Epidemiology and End Results (SEER) database indicate that patients undergoing neoadjuvant radiation therapy had significantly fewer retrieved nodes from the surgical specimen compared with patients undergoing surgery alone after a multivariate analysis. The number of retrieved lymph nodes was significantly higher in patients with N+ disease.[40] This observation of an overall reduction in the number of lymph nodes of patients undergoing neoadjuvant therapy seems to be influenced by the time elapsed between radiation completion and surgical resection. One study showed that the number of recovered lymph nodes was significantly affected by the interval between CRT completion and surgery, but

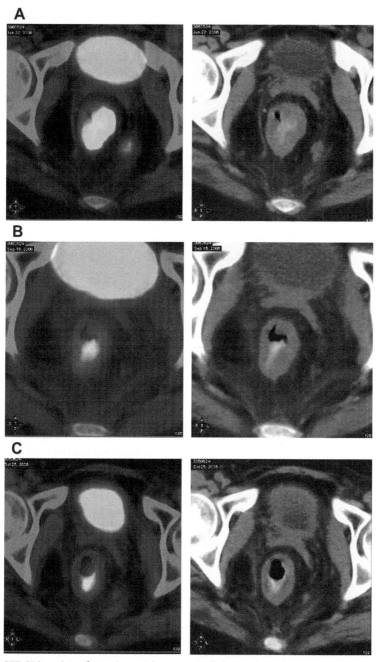

Fig. 3. PET-CT imaging of a patient with a posteriorly located rectal cancer and positive perirectal nodal uptake (*A1, A2*) and incomplete tumor regression after CRT completion as determined by residual rectal uptake within the rectal wall despite no residual nodal uptake at 6 (*B1, B2*) and 12 weeks (*C1, C2*) from CRT.

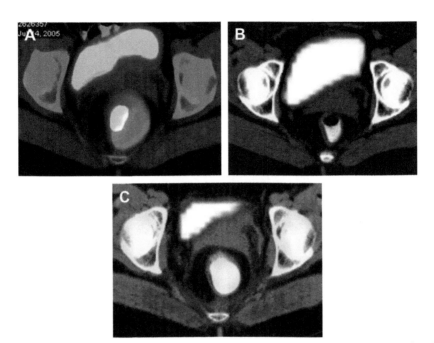

Fig. 4. PET-CT imaging of a patient with a rectal cancer within the right lateral wall (*A*) and complete tumor regression after CRT completion as determined by no residual uptake within the rectal wall at 6 (*B*) and 12 weeks (*C*) from CRT.

not by total radiation doses delivered. Exposure to longer interval periods led to recovery of fewer lymph nodes in patients surgical specimens.[41] This observation has 2 implications: first, the critical and required number of lymph nodes for proper staging of rectal cancer may not be the same for patients undergoing neoadjuvant CRT as for patients who go straight to surgery; second, the effects of radiation on lymph nodes seem to be time dependent, similarly to what has been observed for primary tumor regression.[41] Lymph node recovery may be further influenced by technical issues, including the use of fat-clearing solutions. In this setting, even though fat cleansing solutions were once considered too labor-intensive and potentially toxic, this technique may ultimately result in improvement in rectal cancer staging in patients undergoing neoadjuvant CRT.[42]

In a retrospective review of patients with incomplete clinical response after neoadjuvant CRT, the outcomes of patients with no recovered nodes in the radical surgery specimen were slightly better than those of patients with node-negative disease, and significantly better than patients with node-positive disease. These findings suggest that patients with an absence of nodes in the resected specimen may represent a subset of patients with particularly increased sensitivity to CRT.[43]

The risk of lymph node micrometastases also seems to be decreased in patients after neoadjuvant CRT. Even so, the concept of nodal sterilization secondary to neoadjuvant CRT remains highly controversial. The finding of mucin deposits within lymph nodes that have no residual cancer cells in patients with rectal cancer who have received neoadjuvant CRT provides indirect evidence of such sterilization.[44] More recently, a single-institution experience has reported the presence of acellullar mucin in up to 27% of specimens with ypCR. Among these, 19% showed acellular mucin within the nodes recovered after radical resection. The presence of acellular mucin within the specimen had no negative influence on the outcomes of these patients, suggesting that this may represent evidence of tumor sterilization both within the rectum and the lymph nodes.[45]

One of the main concerns after neoadjuvant CRT is that, even though the primary tumor may have completely regressed, there is still a risk of residual node positivity. The rates of nodal disease (N+) in patients with complete primary tumor regression (ypT0) vary between 0% and 7%.[46–49] Again, these rates might reflect differences in timing of surgery and doses of radiation therapy. Coincidentally, the higher rates of ypT0N+ are consistently associated with patients undergoing surgery 6 weeks after CRT completion and could represent lymph node metastases that are in the process of regressing. In addition, the clinical relevance of microscopic residual lymph node metastases is still poorly understood. In a parallel to colorectal cancer, the presence of lymph node micrometastases has not been completely accepted as a clinically relevant finding.[46,50] Even in the worst-case scenario, the risk of residual microscopic lymph node metastases after ypT0 is still less than the risk of residual microscopic lymph node metastases in patients with pT1 rectal cancer, around 12% to 13%, and is frequently managed by transanal local excision alone.[51]

In this setting, patients without microscopic residual disease would potentially not benefit from radical surgery. Instead, surgery would unnecessarily expose them to immediate morbidity and mortality as well as the consequence of permanent or temporary stomas. Moreover, radical rectal resection may lead to functional disabilities, including fecal incontinence, as well as urinary and sexual dysfunction.

The finding of ypCR in up to 42% of cases raised the question regarding the benefits of such a surgery if not a single cancer cell is removed.[15,16] For these reasons, an alternative approach was suggested in highly selected patients with complete clinical response. With this alternative approach, patients with no clinical or radiological signs of residual disease at least 8 weeks after CRT completion would be managed by no immediate surgery.[16]

The Watch-and-wait Protocol Algorithm

Patients with complete clinical response, either after clinical assessment or after transanal local excision (ypT0), are enrolled in a strict follow-up program (**Fig. 5**).[52] Adherence to the follow-up program is critical because distinguishing between complete and near-complete responses may be difficult. This algorithm includes monthly follow-up visits with digital rectal examination and rigid proctoscopy in every visit for the first 12 months. CEA levels are determined every 2 months. As discussed previously, PET-CT is currently being investigated for its usefulness in tumor response assessment in a prospective study. Other radiological studies, such as pelvic CT scans or magnetic resonance imaging, are performed at the time of initial tumor response assessment, and then every 6 months if there are no signs of tumor recurrence. The main objective of these radiological studies is to rule out any sign of residual extrarectal disease, such as residual nodal disease that would require further investigation or even radical resection.

Patients are fully informed that complete clinical regression of their primary tumor may be temporary and disease recurrence or tumor regrowth may occur at any time during follow-up. In the case of obvious recurrence or tumor regrowth, radical surgery is strongly recommended. Small nodules or scars may develop over time and can be managed by full-thickness transanal excision (either standard or endoscopic microsurgery), primarily as a diagnostic approach.

After 1 year of sustained, complete clinical response, patients are recommended for follow-up visits every 3 months, using the same clinical assessment tools mentioned

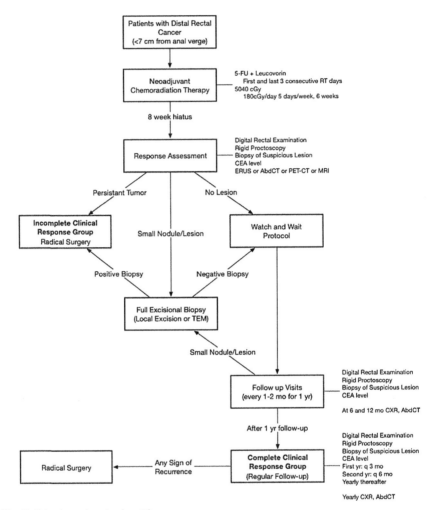

Fig. 5. Watch-and-wait algorithm.

earlier. This arbitrary 12-month period has been suggested by us as a period long enough for one to decide and classify patients as having a complete, incomplete, or near-complete response. This treatment strategy evolved since the beginning of our experience in 1991, and, with time, our accuracy in clinical assessment and judgment has significantly improved. Earlier, patients were more frequently followed without immediate surgery after a near-complete clinical response with the hope that time would lead to a complete clinical response. More recently, these patients have been more readily assessed using full-thickness local excision as a diagnostic procedure, and are then either managed by strict observation or referred to immediate radical surgery.

Long-term Results

Even though no immediate surgery was considered an alternative approach at our institution, most patients were still managed by radical surgery, particularly patients with incomplete clinical response and those in situations in which residual cancer could not be ruled out. These situations include patients with residual scars that were not amenable to local excision and patients with partial narrowing of the rectum impeding rectal visualization. In this setting, several patients ultimately underwent radical surgery and were found to have ypCR after pathologic examination.

Patients with complete clinical response who were managed nonoperatively were compared with patients with ypCR to understand the benefits of radical surgery in both survival and local disease control.[53] Patients managed by observation alone oncologically fared no worse than patients managed by radical surgery. Systemic recurrence rates and long-term survival were similar. Local recurrence was higher in the group of patients managed nonoperatively. These local failures were all restricted to the rectal wall, all were amenable to salvage therapy, and no pelvic relapse was observed.

Long-term results of patients were also compared with final disease stage. Survival of patients was closely associated with final (clinical or pathologic) staging. As described earlier, patients with clinically complete response (stage c0) had similar long-term results to patients with ypCR (stage p0). Also, these survival rates were significantly better than those observed for patients with stage ypII and ypIII. Patients with stage ypI had intermediate long-term survival rates.

These results suggest that, in the absence of any benefit in overall and disease-free survival, no immediate surgery after a complete clinical response might be superior to immediate radical surgery by avoiding potential unnecessary immediate morbidity, mortality, sexual and urinary dysfunctions, and the requirement for temporary or definitive stomas.

Survival and Recurrence

Prospective randomized studies have failed to demonstrate a survival benefit in patients undergoing neoadjuvant CRT compared with adjuvant CRT. One possible explanation could be the detrimental effect of neoadjuvant CRT on host immunologic response against rectal cancer, such as the potential blockade of peritumoral inflammatory and immunologic response.[54,55]

However, it has recently been shown that the addition of adjuvant chemotherapy can improve survival in highly selected patients with increased local tumor downstaging after neoadjuvant CRT (ypT0-2).[56] These results may lead to a significant change in management of these patients, who used to be considered for adjuvant therapy according to pretreatment staging (stage cIII) or according to final pathologic staging (only in the presence of ypN+ disease). In this setting, there is a chance that patients with complete clinical response might experience additional benefits in survival after receiving adjuvant systemic therapy.

In our data, systemic recurrences in patients with complete clinical response managed nonoperatively did occur considerably earlier during follow-up than local recurrences.[17] Besides intrinsic tumor behavior, this may be partly explained by the limitations in current imaging modalities to detect microscopic foci of metastatic disease at initial presentation. Again, in this particular series of patients, adjuvant systemic therapy was considered only in patients with stage ypIII disease.[17]

Local recurrences may occur in nearly 10% of these patients managed nonoperatively after a complete clinical response. So far, in all of these patients, local recurrences have been exclusively detected within the rectal wall. There have been no extrarectal pelvic recurrences in this experience. In addition, even though some recurrences within the rectal wall may develop deep in the outer layers of the bowel, in all cases there was some expression of such recurrence through the lumen that could be detected by clinical assessment. Therefore, these recurrences or regrowths may develop from microscopic residual foci in the outer layers of the rectum and should be detected by clinical assessment, given the close follow-up and rigorous examination schedule (**Fig. 6**).

Local recurrences developed later in follow-up than those in patients who undergo radical surgery alone. This finding has also been observed in other series, in which more than one-third of patients who developed local recurrences after neoadjuvant CRT and radical surgery did so after 5 years of follow-up. In contrast, more than 75% of patients who develop local recurrences after radical surgery alone do so within 2 years of follow-up. Besides improved understanding of tumor behavior after CRT, the likelihood of late recurrences may have additional implications in terms of long-term follow-up and surveillance strategies in these patients.

Final pathologic features are the most important prognostic factors for survival in patients undergoing neoadjuvant CRT for rectal cancer as opposed to initial (pre-CRT) staging.[57] This observation supports the excellent survival outcomes of patients with complete clinical response, comparable with patients with ypCR observed in our experience.[58] It also suggests that final management of these patients should probably be determined and tailored according to response to neoadjuvant CRT.

Salvage Therapy

It is significant that all local recurrences after nonoperative treatment of patients with complete clinical response following neoadjuvant CRT were amenable to salvage therapy. In our experience, these recurrences and their salvage procedures were performed at a long interval after CRT completion (mean interval >50 months) and included abdomino-perineal (APR) in almost half of these patients. Almost one-third of these patients presented with considerably low and superficial recurrences, amenable to full-thickness transanal excision. In these patients, APR was refused because a definitive surgical alternative and local excision was performed.[17]

There was a significant subset of patients who developed early tumor regrowth, within the initial arbitrary 12-month probation period after suspicion of complete clinical response and no immediate surgery. These patients were most likely misdiagnosed for complete clinical response and had their definitive surgical resection postponed or delayed for a variable period of time. The issue was raised on whether these patients could have been harmed from the oncological point of view, including recurrence and long-term survival. However, these patients did no worse than patients with incomplete clinical response detected immediately and managed by radical surgery 8 weeks after

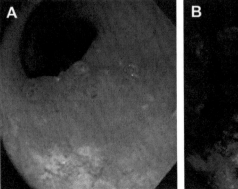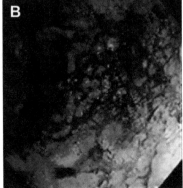

Fig. 6. Endoscopic view of a local recurrence after initial complete clinical response; (A) standard view and (B) view after Nankin ink injection.

CRT completion. The patients initially suspected for complete clinical response and who underwent delayed surgery presented with significantly earlier pathologic staging (including lower rates of positive lymph node metastases), further supporting the idea that downstaging is a time-dependent phenomenon. In addition, these patients were more frequently managed by APR. This could partially reflect a motivation by the surgeon and the patient to delay the final decision for surgery until a later response assessment, knowing that tumor regression could still proceed. The exact time for the surgeon to decide whether surgery should be performed is still unknown. Available data suggest that, in patients with high suspicion for complete clinical response, waiting more than the usual 8 weeks brings no harm to these patients.[52]

Perspectives

Several aspects in the management of complete clinical response after neoadjuvant CRT remain unresolved and should be a focus of future clinical and molecular genetics research.

An area of significant interest is the development of novel radiation therapy regimens including alternative radiation doses, delivery methods, and technical variants to maximize radiation-related tumor cell death and minimize side effects. In addition, the search for improved chemotherapy regimens might lead to an increase in the rate of complete clinical response and, possibly, improved survival rates. For these reasons, some investigators have suggested the use of aggressive induction chemotherapy before the delivery of radiation to provide immediate treatment of undetected microscopic foci of metastatic tumor cells in addition to the primary tumor.[59] These regimens are currently under investigation in controlled trials to provide data on safety and long-term benefits. Another strategy involving the use of alternative chemotherapy regimens in neoadjuvant CRT is the delivery of chemotherapy during the waiting or resting period between radiation completion and tumor response assessment. Our group has recently analyzed the outcomes of a small series of patients being managed by this novel extended CRT regimen consisting of 54 Gy of radiation delivered in 180 Gy/d fractions and 5-FU/leucovorin-based chemotherapy delivered in 3 cycles during radiation therapy and in 3 additional cycles during the resting period after radiation completion (all cycles given every 21 days). The sustained complete clinical response rate (>12 months) was 65% in the series including T2/T3 distal rectal cancers, with no significant increase in chemotherapy-related toxicity rates. After a recent update of this same series of patients, complete clinical response rates seem to be sustained after a median follow-up of more than 36 months at 65%.[60]

The greatest challenge in rectal cancer management will be the incorporation of molecular biology information into clinical practice, potentially allowing clinicians and surgeons to identify patients with increased likelihood of tumor downsizing, downstaging, or even complete pathologic regression after neoadjuvant CRT. In one study using DNA microarray, a set of 95 genes allowed the identification of patients who would develop ypCR after neoadjuvant CRT and radical surgery with 85% accuracy. Future studies, including direct gene sequencing with newly developed sequencing technologies, may attempt to identify a subset of genes capable of identifying which patients are most likely to undergo a complete clinical response after neoadjuvant CRT, thus avoiding radical surgery in a significant number of patients.[61]

REFERENCES

1. Sauer R, Becker H, Hohenberger W, et al. Preoperative versus postoperative chemoradiotherapy for rectal cancer. N Engl J Med 2004;351(17):1731–40.

2. Folkesson J, Birgisson H, Pahlman L, et al. Swedish rectal cancer trial: long lasting benefits from radiotherapy on survival and local recurrence rate. J Clin Oncol 2005;23(24):5644–50.

3. Kapiteijn E, Marijnen CA, Nagtegaal ID, et al. Preoperative radiotherapy combined with total mesorectal excision for resectable rectal cancer. N Engl J Med 2001;345(9):638–46.

4. Peeters KC, Marijnen CA, Nagtegaal ID, et al. The TME trial after a median follow-up of 6 years: increased local control but no survival benefit in irradiated patients with resectable rectal carcinoma. Ann Surg 2007;246(5):693–701.

5. Tjandra JJ, Kilkenny JW, Buie WD, et al. Practice parameters for the management of rectal cancer (revised). Dis Colon Rectum 2005;48(3):411–23.

6. Habr-Gama A, Perez RO, Kiss DR, et al. Preoperative chemoradiation therapy for low rectal cancer. Impact on downstaging and sphincter-saving operations. Hepatogastroenterology 2004;51(60):1703–7.

7. Guillem JG, Diaz-Gonzalez JA, Minsky BD, et al. cT3N0 rectal cancer: potential overtreatment with preoperative chemoradiotherapy is warranted. J Clin Oncol 2008;26(3):368–73.

8. Petersen S, Hellmich G, von Mildenstein K, et al. Is surgery-only the adequate treatment approach for T2N0 rectal cancer? J Surg Oncol 2006;93(5):350–4.

9. Rengan R, Paty P, Wong WD, et al. Distal cT2N0 rectal cancer: is there an alternative to abdominoperineal resection? J Clin Oncol 2005;23(22):4905–12.

10. Chessin DB, Enker W, Cohen AM, et al. Complications after preoperative combined modality therapy and radical resection of locally advanced rectal cancer: a 14-year experience from a specialty service. J Am Coll Surg 2005; 200(6):876–82 [discussion: 882–4].

11. Eriksen MT, Wibe A, Norstein J, et al. Anastomotic leakage following routine mesorectal excision for rectal cancer in a national cohort of patients. Colorectal Dis 2005;7(1):51–7.

12. Matthiessen P, Hallbook O, Andersson M, et al. Risk factors for anastomotic leakage after anterior resection of the rectum. Colorectal Dis 2004;6(6):462–9.

13. Perez RO, Habr-Gama A, Seid VE, et al. Loop ileostomy morbidity: timing of closure matters. Dis Colon Rectum 2006;49(10):1539–45.

14. Greene FL, American Joint Committee on Cancer, American Cancer Society. AJCC cancer staging manual. 6th edition. New York: Springer-Verlag; 2002.

15. Sanghera P, Wong DW, McConkey CC, et al. Chemoradiotherapy for rectal cancer: an updated analysis of factors affecting pathological response. Clin Oncol (R Coll Radiol) 2008;20(2):176–83.

16. Habr-Gama A, de Souza PM, Ribeiro U Jr, et al. Low rectal cancer: impact of radiation and chemotherapy on surgical treatment. Dis Colon Rectum 1998;41(9): 1087–96.

17. Habr-Gama A, Perez RO, Proscurshim I, et al. Patterns of failure and survival for nonoperative treatment of stage c0 distal rectal cancer following neoadjuvant chemoradiation therapy. J Gastrointest Surg 2006;10(10):1319–28 [discussion: 1328–9].

18. Tulchinsky H, Shmueli E, Figer A, et al. An interval >7 weeks between neoadjuvant therapy and surgery improves pathologic complete response and disease-free survival in patients with locally advanced rectal cancer. Ann Surg Oncol 2008;15(10):2661–7.

19. Moore HG, Gittleman AE, Minsky BD, et al. Rate of pathologic complete response with increased interval between preoperative combined modality therapy and rectal cancer resection. Dis Colon Rectum 2004;47(3):279–86.

20. Kalady MF, de Campos-Lobato LF, Stocchi L, et al. Predictive factors of patho-
    logic complete response after neoadjuvant chemoradiation for rectal cancer.
    Ann Surg 2009;250(4):582–9.
21. Withers HR, Haustermans K. Where next with preoperative radiation therapy for
    rectal cancer? Int J Radiat Oncol Biol Phys 2004;58(2):597–602.
22. Kerr SF, Norton S, Glynne-Jones R. Delaying surgery after neoadjuvant chemora-
    diotherapy for rectal cancer may reduce postoperative morbidity without compro-
    mising prognosis. Br J Surg 2008;95(12):1534–40.
23. Hiotis SP, Weber SM, Cohen AM, et al. Assessing the predictive value of clinical
    complete response to neoadjuvant therapy for rectal cancer: an analysis of 488
    patients. J Am Coll Surg 2002;194(2):131–5 [discussion: 135–6].
24. Park YA, Lee KY, Kim NK, et al. Prognostic effect of perioperative change of
    serum carcinoembryonic antigen level: a useful tool for detection of systemic
    recurrence in rectal cancer. Ann Surg Oncol 2006;13(5):645–50.
25. Das P, Skibber JM, Rodriguez-Bigas MA, et al. Predictors of tumor response and
    downstaging in patients who receive preoperative chemoradiation for rectal
    cancer. Cancer 2007;109(9):1750–5.
26. Moreno Garcia V, Cejas P, Blanco Codesido M, et al. Prognostic value of carci-
    noembryonic antigen level in rectal cancer treated with neoadjuvant chemoradio-
    therapy. Int J Colorectal Dis 2009;24(7):741–8.
27. Perez RO, Sao Juliao GP, Habr-Gama A, et al. The role of carcinoembriogenic
    antigen in predicting response and survival to neoadjuvant chemoradiotherapy
    for distal rectal cancer. Dis Colon Rectum 2009;52(6):1137–43.
28. Brown G. Staging rectal cancer: endoscopic ultrasound and pelvic MRI. Cancer
    Imaging 2008;8(Suppl A):S43–5.
29. Koh DM, Chau I, Tait D, et al. Evaluating mesorectal lymph nodes in rectal
    cancer before and after neoadjuvant chemoradiation using thin-section T2-
    weighted magnetic resonance imaging. Int J Radiat Oncol Biol Phys 2008;
    71(2):456–61.
30. Shihab OC, Moran BJ, Heald RJ, et al. MRI staging of low rectal cancer. Eur Ra-
    diol 2008;19(3):643–50.
31. Mezzi G, Arcidiacono PG, Carrara S, et al. Endoscopic ultrasound and magnetic
    resonance imaging for re-staging rectal cancer after radiotherapy. World J Gas-
    troenterol 2009;15(44):5563–7.
32. Suppiah A, Hunter IA, Cowley J, et al. Magnetic resonance imaging accuracy in
    assessing tumour down-staging following chemoradiation in rectal cancer. Colo-
    rectal Dis 2009;11(3):249–53.
33. Calvo FA, Domper M, Matute R, et al. 18F-FDG positron emission tomography
    staging and restaging in rectal cancer treated with preoperative chemoradiation.
    Int J Radiat Oncol Biol Phys 2004;58(2):528–35.
34. Guillem JG, Puig-La Calle J Jr, Akhurst T, et al. Prospective assessment of
    primary rectal cancer response to preoperative radiation and chemotherapy
    using 18-fluorodeoxyglucose positron emission tomography. Dis Colon Rectum
    2000;43(1):18–24.
35. Guillem JG, Moore HG, Akhurst T, et al. Sequential preoperative fluorodeoxyglu-
    cose-positron emission tomography assessment of response to preoperative
    chemoradiation: a means for determining longterm outcomes of rectal cancer.
    J Am Coll Surg 2004;199(1):1–7.
36. Chessin DB, Kiran RP, Akhurst T, et al. The emerging role of 18F-fluorodeoxyglu-
    cose positron emission tomography in the management of primary and recurrent
    rectal cancer. J Am Coll Surg 2005;201(6):948–56.

37. Kristiansen C, Loft A, Berthelsen AK, et al. PET/CT and histopathologic response to preoperative chemoradiation therapy in locally advanced rectal cancer. Dis Colon Rectum 2008;51(1):21–5.

38. Habr-Gama A, Gama-Rodrigues J, Perez RO, et al. Late assessment of local control by PET in patients with distal rectal cancer managed non-operatively after complete tumor regression following neoadjuvant chemoradiation. Tech Coloproctol 2008;12(1):74–6.

39. Kumar PP, Good RR, Plantz SH, et al. Technique of postoperative pelvic radiation in the management of rectal and rectosigmoid carcinoma. J Natl Med Assoc 1987;79(6):609–15.

40. Baxter NN, Morris AM, Rothenberger DA, et al. Impact of preoperative radiation for rectal cancer on subsequent lymph node evaluation: a population-based analysis. Int J Radiat Oncol Biol Phys 2005;61(2):426–31.

41. Sermier A, Gervaz P, Egger JF, et al. Lymph node retrieval in abdominoperineal surgical specimen is radiation time-dependent. World J Surg Oncol 2006;4:29.

42. Wang H, Safar B, Wexner SD, et al. The clinical significance of fat clearance lymph node harvest for invasive rectal adenocarcinoma following neoadjuvant therapy. Dis Colon Rectum 2009;52(10):1767–73.

43. Habr-Gama A, Perez RO, Proscurshim I, et al. Absence of lymph nodes in the resected specimen after radical surgery for distal rectal cancer and neoadjuvant chemoradiation therapy: what does it mean? Dis Colon Rectum 2008;51(3): 277–83.

44. Perez RO, Bresciani BH, Bresciani C, et al. Mucinous colorectal adenocarcinoma: influence of mucin expression (Muc1, 2 and 5) on clinico-pathological features and prognosis. Int J Colorectal Dis 2008;23(8):757–65.

45. Smith KD, Tan D, Das P, et al. Clinical significance of acellular mucin in rectal adenocarcinoma patients with a pathologic complete response to preoperative chemoradiation. Ann Surg 2010;251(2):261–4.

46. Perez RO, Habr-Gama A, Nishida Arazawa ST, et al. Lymph node micrometastasis in stage II distal rectal cancer following neoadjuvant chemoradiation therapy. Int J Colorectal Dis 2005;20(5):434–9.

47. Stipa F, Zernecke A, Moore HG, et al. Residual mesorectal lymph node involvement following neoadjuvant combined-modality therapy: rationale for radical resection? Ann Surg Oncol 2004;11(2):187–91.

48. Pucciarelli S, Capirci C, Emanuele U, et al. Relationship between pathologic T-stage and nodal metastasis after preoperative chemoradiotherapy for locally advanced rectal cancer. Ann Surg Oncol 2005;12(2):111–6.

49. Zmora O, Dasilva GM, Gurland B, et al. Does rectal wall tumor eradication with preoperative chemoradiation permit a change in the operative strategy? Dis Colon Rectum 2004;47(10):1607–12.

50. Fleming FJ, Hayanga AJ, Glynn F, et al. Incidence and prognostic influence of lymph node micrometastases in rectal cancer. Eur J Surg Oncol 2007;33(8): 998–1002.

51. Nascimbeni R, Burgart LJ, Nivatvongs S, et al. Risk of lymph node metastasis in T1 carcinoma of the colon and rectum. Dis Colon Rectum 2002;45(2):200–6.

52. Habr-Gama A, Perez RO, Proscurshim I, et al. Interval between surgery and neoadjuvant chemoradiation therapy for distal rectal cancer: does delayed surgery have an impact on outcome? Int J Radiat Oncol Biol Phys 2008;71(4):1181–8.

53. Habr-Gama A, Perez RO, Nadalin W, et al. Operative versus nonoperative treatment for stage 0 distal rectal cancer following chemoradiation therapy: long-term results. Ann Surg 2004;240(4):711–7 [discussion: 717–8].

54. Wichmann MW, Meyer G, Adam M, et al. Detrimental immunologic effects of preoperative chemoradiotherapy in advanced rectal cancer. Dis Colon Rectum 2003;46(7):875–87.
55. Perez RO, Habr-Gama A, dos Santos RM, et al. Peritumoral inflammatory infiltrate is not a prognostic factor in distal rectal cancer following neoadjuvant chemoradiation therapy. J Gastrointest Surg 2007;11(11):1534–40.
56. Collette L, Bosset JF, den Dulk M, et al. Patients with curative resection of cT3-4 rectal cancer after preoperative radiotherapy or radiochemotherapy: does anybody benefit from adjuvant fluorouracil-based chemotherapy? A trial of the European Organisation for Research and Treatment of Cancer Radiation Oncology Group. J Clin Oncol 2007;25(28):4379–86.
57. Quah HM, Chou JF, Gonen M, et al. Pathologic stage is most prognostic of disease-free survival in locally advanced rectal cancer patients after preoperative chemoradiation. Cancer 2008;113(1):57–64.
58. Habr-Gama A, Perez RO, Nadalin W, et al. Long-term results of preoperative chemoradiation for distal rectal cancer correlation between final stage and survival. J Gastrointest Surg 2005;9(1):90–9 [discussion: 99–101].
59. Chau I, Brown G, Cunningham D, et al. Neoadjuvant capecitabine and oxaliplatin followed by synchronous chemoradiation and total mesorectal excision in magnetic resonance imaging-defined poor-risk rectal cancer. J Clin Oncol 2006;24(4):668–74.
60. Habr-Gama A, Perez RO, Sabbaga J, et al. Increasing the rates of complete response to neoadjuvant chemoradiotherapy for distal rectal cancer: results of a prospective study using additional chemotherapy during the resting period. Dis Colon Rectum 2009;52(12):1927–34.
61. Kim IJ, Lim SB, Kang HC, et al. Microarray gene expression profiling for predicting complete response to preoperative chemoradiotherapy in patients with advanced rectal cancer. Dis Colon Rectum 2007;50(9):1342–53.

Multidisciplinary Approach to Recurrent/ Unresectable Rectal Cancer: How to Prepare for the Extent of Resection

Miguel A. Rodriguez-Bigas, MD*, George J. Chang, MD,
John M. Skibber, MD

KEYWORDS
- Recurrent rectal cancer • Intraoperative radiation
- Pelvic exenteration • Abdominosacral resection

Despite advances in surgical techniques and the use of chemoradiation, local recurrence is still a significant problem in the management of cancer of the rectum. Locally recurrent rectal cancer (LRRC) can be debilitating and potentially lead to a poor quality of life (QOL). In the last decade, the incidence of local recurrence after curative resection for rectal cancer has been reported to be between 5% and 17%.[1-8] At the time of diagnosis, approximately 50% of the patients with LRRC will have metastatic disease, but between 30% and 50% of patients will die with local disease alone.[7,9-11] Prognosis among patients with LRRC can be poor because the majority of these patients will not be candidates for salvage surgical resection. The median survival in untreated patients has been reported to be about 8 months.[12] Radiotherapy with or without chemotherapy increases survival to about 11 to 15 months. With aggressive multimodality therapy, for LRRC, the overall 5-year survival rate is 25% to 54%, with higher survival rates for those patients resected with negative margins.[7,13-16] In this article, the multidisciplinary approach to the management of patients with recurrent rectal cancer is discussed.

Department of Surgical Oncology, The University of Texas M.D. Anderson Cancer Center, 1515 Holcombe, Unit 444, Houston, TX 77030, USA
* Corresponding author.
E-mail address: mrodbig@mdanderson.org

Surg Oncol Clin N Am 19 (2010) 847–859
doi:10.1016/j.soc.2010.07.001
1055-3207/10/$ – see front matter © 2010 Elsevier Inc. All rights reserved.

surgonc.theclinics.com

CLINICAL PRESENTATION

The vast majority of local recurrences occur within the first 2 to 3 years after curative surgery.[17,18] Nevertheless, local recurrence can occur after longer intervals. In fact, in patients treated with local excision with or without chemoradiation, local recurrences have been reported at intervals of more than 6 years after primary treatment.[19,20] The majority of patients who develop local recurrence will be symptomatic. The most common symptoms include new onset of pelvic or perineal pain, change in bowel habits, rectal bleeding, and urinary symptoms. In patients who have undergone an abdominoperineal resection, a nonhealing wound could be a sign of locally recurrent disease.

EVALUATION AND IMAGING

For the group of patients who may be candidates for potential surgical resection, careful staging and treatment planning should be performed by a multidisciplinary team. This team includes the surgeon, medical oncologist, radiation oncologist, urologist, plastic and reconstructive surgeon, radiologist, pathologist, enterostomal nurses, social workers, and at times a psychiatrist. A thorough evaluation should be performed to select patients in whom a complete surgical resection can be achieved with negative margins, because these patients will be the ones most likely to benefit. Surgical salvage procedures for LRRC include en bloc resection of adjacent organs or structures, such as total pelvic exenterations (TPE) and abdominosacral resection (AR), which are highly morbid, and thus could lead to worse quality of life for patients than symptomatic management.

A careful history and physical examination should be performed. In patients presenting with pain, the quality and characteristics of the pain are important in determining the potential for resectability. Patients with LRRC presenting with pain radiating to the back of the leg will most likely have involvement of the sciatic nerve and most likely will not be amenable to resection as opposed to patients presenting with just pelvic discomfort. It is important to elicit symptoms and signs regarding adjacent structures, such as pneumaturia, fecaluria, vaginal bleeding, abdominal pain with cramps, recurrent fever or chills, and weight loss, among others. Once a careful history has been taken, a physical examination, including rectal and vaginal examination and proctoscopy (in those patients who have had a sphincter-saving procedure), should be performed. This examination will allow evaluation for whether or not the recurrence is fixed, and may give the clinician an idea of the extent of the recurrence, such as involvement of the bladder or prostate, vagina, perineum, and on occasion metastatic disease to the groins. An effort should be made to obtain prior medical records, including operative reports, radiation therapy treatment plans and dosage given, as well as documentation regarding chemotherapy administered. As discussed later, patients with LRRC are candidates for reirradiation, and thus, prior radiotherapy records are important in planning re-treatment. At times it is difficult to evaluate patients in the office or clinic setting, and thus, an examination under anesthesia is necessary. In the authors' practice, every effort is made to tissue document a local recurrence before embarking in the multimodality treatment of a local recurrence.

Evaluation of patients with locally recurrent rectal cancer should include
 History and physical examination (obtain previous medical records, including operative reports, radiation schedule and portals, and chemotherapy schedules)
 Proctoscopy
 Colonoscopy

Imaging
    Computerized axial tomography (CAT)
    MRI
    Positron emission tomography (PET)
    Positron emission tomography and CAT scan (PET/CT).

IMAGING

To adequately stage patients with LRRC, once the initial evaluation is completed, imaging studies are performed. Although some investigators have advocated endorectal ultrasound (EUS) in patients with LRRC after local excision, the authors have not been able to demonstrate its utility in routine practice.[8] EUS can be useful to perform needle-guided biopsy of a pelvic recurrence. CAT and MRI scans should be used to evaluate patients. The authors usually start evaluating patients with a CAT scan of the chest, abdomen, and pelvis. The advantage of doing this is that not only will local disease information be provided but distant disease can be identified. A pelvic MRI provides improved ability to distinguish posttreatment changes from viable tumor in comparison to CT imaging and provides excellent detail of surrounding pelvic structures, including sacral nerve roots, major pelvic vasculature, and bone, all of which are the parameters that need to be evaluated to determine resectability. It is important to note that with both of these modalities, the extent of involvement by the LRRC may be underestimated. Although not routinely part of the initial surgical staging, positron emission tomography fused with CAT scan (PET/CT) is employed in those cases where equivocal radiographic evidence of both local and distant disease is present. PET/CT has been reported to change the management in up to 14% of patients with LRRC.[8,21]

CLASSIFICATION OF THE RECURRENCE

Several classifications have been proposed for LRRC.[10,22–24] The purpose of these classifications has been to define the structures that the LRRC involves, assess resectability, plan the extent of resection, and compare outcomes.[15] The Mayo Clinic classification relies on the degree of fixation of the recurrence, and encompasses the earliest type of recurrences with no fixation to advanced recurrence with 3 or more points of fixation.[10] Wanebo and colleagues[22] proposed a classification based on modified criteria from the TNM staging system. In this classification, recurrences are described as local/minimal (within the bowel wall) to extensive invasion of the pelvis, including bony structures and sidewall.[22] Yamada and colleagues[23] classified the recurrences as localized, sacral invasive, and lateral invasive types and correlated survival with each type. None of the subjects with a lateral invasive recurrence survived 5 years.[23] The Memorial Sloan Kettering classification is based on the anatomic location of the recurrence.[24]

In the authors' experience, the classification of recurrences based on anatomic location is clinically most useful. In general, anastomotic (after low anterior resections and transanal excisions), inferior or perineal recurrences, and central recurrences (those involving the rectum or urogenital organs) are the most amenable to surgical salvage. Posterior recurrences are also amenable to surgical salvage when sacral involvement remains below the second sacral vertebrae (S2). Lateral recurrences are the most difficult to address because involvement of the lateral bony pelvic structures, the major blood vessels, and other lateral structures may preclude a resection with negative margins.

SURGICAL PLANNING

Once patients have been evaluated and the images reviewed, a thorough and frank discussion between the surgeon and patients regarding the options for treatment and the expected treatment outcomes is essential. In addition, presentation at a tumor board or a multidisciplinary conference to discuss the options of treatment is preferred. It must be understood that whenever surgery is being considered, imaging is only one part of the decision making process. Many factors need to be considered in the decision-making process, including the general status of patients, the physical findings, the available treatment options, the biology or aggressiveness of the disease, and the patients' opinion. The following list demonstrates nonresectability criteria for locally recurrent rectal cancer. **Fig. 1** illustrates 2 examples of unresectable recurrences; whereas, **Fig. 2** shows a posterior recurrence and its reconstruction after an abdominosacral resection.

Preoperative criteria for nonresectability of locally recurrent rectal cancer
  Anatomic
  Involvement

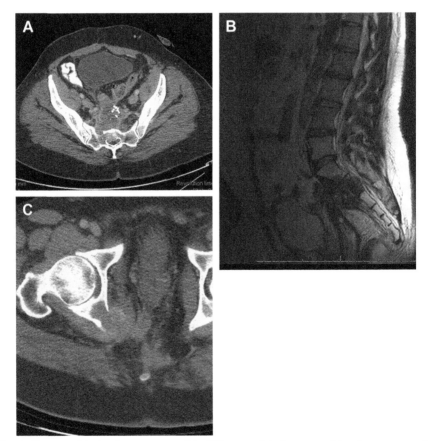

Fig. 1. Unresectable local recurrences. (*A*) CAT scan axial view central local recurrence. (*B*) MRI sagittal view same patient recurrence involving S1–2. (*C*) CAT scan axial view of lateral recurrence involving sciatic notch.

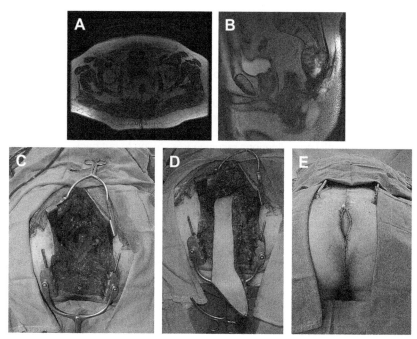

Fig. 2. Resectable local recurrence. (*A*) MRI axial view of locally recurrent rectal cancer at level of S3. (*B*) MRI sagittal view of locally recurrent rectal cancer at level of S3. (*C*) Defect after abdominosacral resection. (*D*) Vertical rectus abdominis flap to cover defect. (*Courtesy of* Patrick Garvey, MD, MD Anderson Cancer Center, Department of Plastic and Reconstructive Surgery, Houston, TX.) (*E*) Vertical Rectus Abdominis Flap sutured in place. (*Courtesy of* Patrick Garvey, MD, MD Anderson Cancer Center, Department of Plastic and Reconstructive Surgery, Houston, TX.)

    Above S2 or sacral ala
    Acetabulum
    Common and external iliac arteries
    Sciatic nerve or sciatic notch
    Bilateral hydronephrosis (relative)
Biologic
    Metastatic disease not amenable to resection
    Para-aortic lymph node involvement
Patient
    Poor performance status
    Unacceptable surgical risks because of comorbidities
Technical
    Inability to obtain a negative margin of resection.

If patients are considered to be potentially resectable with negative margins, both the surgeon and patients must understand that imaging is not perfect, and may underestimate the level of invasiveness or adherence by the recurrence. The surgeon must be prepared to remove the tumor and adjacent structures or organs adhered to the tumor. Surgical options for LRRC include local resection of the recurrence, bowel resection with primary anastomosis, abdominoperineal resection, pelvic exenteration, and abdominosacral resection.

In general, surgical resection of LRRC involves a multidisciplinary surgical team. In addition to the primary surgeon, the surgical team may include urologists, gynecologists, plastic and reconstructive surgeons, neurosurgeons, and radiation oncologists. Careful multidisciplinary planning will provide the most satisfactory results. Unfortunately, there are times where in order to intraoperatively assess resectability, the surgeon has to commit to performing the resection without knowing whether or not negative margins will be obtained. The authors' call this the point of no return, and it is not an ideal situation because either microscopic or gross tumor will be left behind. If the procedure can be done with acceptable morbidity, it may indeed be a better situation than the potential complications resulting from trying to put back together structures that have been already severed or violated with the attendant complications and poor quality of life related to those potential complications or tumor-related issues.

Multimodality Therapy for Locally Recurrent Rectal Cancer

Surgery is the mainstay in the management of patients with LRRC. Chances of surgical salvage appear to improve according to the radicality of the primary procedure. In a series from The Netherlands, Dresen and colleagues[25] reported that subjects who had undergone an anterior resection at the time of their primary tumor diagnosis had a 20% higher chance undergoing radical surgery for their LRRC than those subjects who had undergone an abdominoperineal resection at the time of their primary tumor surgery.

The 5-year survival after surgical salvage for LRRC has been reported to range between 18% and 58%.[8,15,26,27] Morbidity has been reported to be between 21% and 82%.[8,15,26] Wound complications have been a major source of morbidity in these patients. The incidence of major wound problems has decreased with the use of myocutaneous flaps. Perioperative mortality has been reported to be up to 8%.[15] With advances in critical care, a multidisciplinary team approach, and specialized centers doing these procedures, mortality has decreased.

The majority of patients with local recurrence will have been treated with chemoradiation in addition to their primary tumor surgery. In those patients who have not been treated with chemoradiation, the latter needs to be considered before surgical salvage. To maximize the effects of chemoradiation, the authors usually wait 6 to 8 weeks before surgery. Valentini and colleagues[28] reported 29% clinical downstaging after reirradiation and an 8.5% complete pathologic response in resected specimens. In that series, the overall response rate (complete response [CR] + partial response [PR]) after chemoradiation for locally recurrent rectal cancer was 44.1%.[28] Das and colleagues[29] reported a 3-year overall survival rate of 66% in 18 of 50 subjects who were re-treated with chemoradiation and underwent surgical resection compared with those who did not.

Patients who have been previously treated with adjuvant or neoadjuvant chemoradiation can be re-treated safely with acceptable acute and late toxicity.[28–30] The authors' have reported their experience in re-treatment in 50 subjects with recurrent rectal cancer. Nearly all subjects received 150 cGy fractions twice a day for a total dose of 39 Gy and 48 of the 50 subjects received concurrent 5-fluorouracil–based chemotherapy. Two subjects developed grade 3 acute toxicity and 13 subjects (26%) developed grade 3 and 4 late toxicity. The most common acute toxicity was nausea and vomiting; whereas, the most common late toxicity was small bowel obstruction.[29] Some subjects developed urinary complications, such as ureteral anastomotic stricture and leak, and vesicovaginal and rectovaginal fistulas.

The goal of surgery is to remove the recurrent tumor with a negative margin. In LRRC, the incidence of R1 and R2 resections after surgical salvage has been reported to be between 40% and 58%.[7,13,14,16,25,31] In the Mayo Clinic series, Hanhloser and colleagues[13] reported on 304 subjects who underwent surgery for LRRC. Of these 304 resections, only 9% were considered extended resections (pelvic exenterations and abdominosacral resections). There were 138 subjects (45%) resected with negative margins. A statistically significant difference was reported in 5-year survival for subjects who underwent R0 resections versus those with R1 and R2 resections of 37% versus 16%, respectively.[13] The investigators concluded that surgical margins were the most significant influence for long-term survival after salvage surgery for LRRC.

In 85 consecutive salvage resections for locally recurrent rectal cancer at M.D. Anderson Cancer Center, R0 was achieved in 76% and the 5-year disease-specific survival, overall survival, and pelvic control rates were 46%, 36%, and 51%, respectively.[31] On multivariate regression, negative predictors of overall survival included an elevated carcinoembryonic antigen level and R1 resection. Additional evaluation of biologic markers, including expression of p53, bcl-2, and ki-67, did not demonstrate associations with survival outcome.

Boyle and colleagues[14] reported on 64 subjects who underwent surgery for LRRC. Seven of 64 subjects (11%) were found to be unresectable despite preoperative workup and imaging. Of the 57 subjects who underwent resection, 24 (42%) had R0 resection, 25 (44%) had R1 resection, and 8 (14%) had R2 resection. The morbidity in this study was 44% and the mortality was 1.6%. A total of 49% of the subjects re-recurred locally. Of these, 50% had had a R0 resection; whereas, 56% of those with re-recurrence had a R1 resection.[14] The median survival for the 63 subjects discharged from the hospital was 33.6 months. The investigators reported that the median survival in subjects with R0 resection was statistically better than those with R1 resection.[14]

Wanebo and colleagues[22] reported on 53 subjects who underwent abdominosacral resections with curative intent for LRRC. In this study, only 8 subjects had positive margins of resection. The 5-year survival was 31% with a 5-year disease-free survival of 23%.[22] The postoperative death rate was 8%, and the morbidity included 20% prolonged intubation, 34% sepsis, and 38% posterior wound or flap separation. The mean blood loss was greater than 8 L, and the total surgical time was approximately 20 hours. The investigators concluded that in well-selected patients, abdominosacral resection can be performed with acceptable morbidity and mortality.[22]

Akasu and colleagues[16] reported on 40 of 44 subjects who underwent abdominosacral resections with curative intent for LRRC, not involving S1 or the bony lateral pelvic sidewall, over a 17-year period. A total of 37 subjects had macroscopic curative resections, including 4 subjects who had metastatic disease resected. Contrary to Wanebo and colleagues, the procedure was performed as a 1-stage procedure and no myocutaneous flaps were used. R0 resection was obtained in 60% of the subjects. The mean operating room time was 7521 minutes and the median estimated blood loss was 3208 mL. The morbidity was 71%, including 10 subjects who required reoperation. The 5-year overall survival was reported to be 34%, with a 24% disease-free survival. Subjects with R2 resections did not survive more than 28 months after the operation. These investigators also reported that subjects with buttock pain had a worse outcome than those subjects with no pain or perineal pain. Subjects presenting with thigh or leg pain did worse than those with buttock pain.[16] In this series, 25 of 37 (68%) subjects who underwent macroscopic curative resection recurred. Fifty-six percent recurred with local and distant disease. None of the re-recurrences were amenable to surgical salvage.[16]

Sagar and colleagues[32] reported on 40 subjects treated with a 2-stage abdominosacral resection for LRRC with curative intent. In 50% of the subjects, a R0 resection was achieved. The morbidity in this study was 60%, with a 30-day mortality of 2.5%.

The mean disease-free interval for subjects with R0 resection was 55.6 months compared with 32.2 months for those with R1 resection. This difference was statistically significant.[32]

INTRAOPERATIVE RADIOTHERAPY

Despite radical surgery for LRRC, local re-recurrence remains a major problem. Thus, in addition to radical surgery, intraoperative radiation therapy (IORT) has been used in an attempt to improve local control. IORT has been reported to yield good local control in primary advanced and recurrent rectal cancer.[11,33] A dose of IORT is about as effective as 2 to 3 times the equivalent fractionated radiotherapy dose.[34,35] IORT can be delivered in 2 ways: (1) by using intraoperative electron beam radiotherapy (IOERT) or (2) by utilizing high-dose rate brachytherapy (HDR-IORT).[36] IOERT will treat depths greater than 1 cm with a choice of electron energies and quick delivery of the radiation.[36] HDR-IORT uses a flexible template, thus allowing to treat all surfaces with concentrating the highest dose in the area at risk.[37] **Fig. 3** illustrates an HDR-IORT

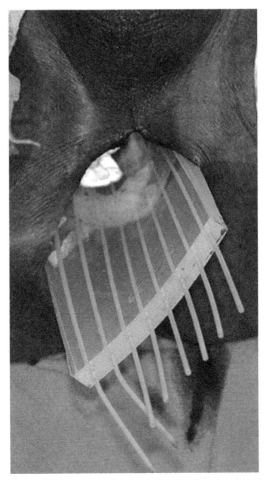

Fig. 3. High-dose rate brachytherapy catheters with template in place before treatment.

template in place. A disadvantage of HDR-IORT is that the time of the treatment depends on the size of the area to be treated and the half-life of the source. There have been no randomized trials with IORT.[36] The indications for IORT vary from center to center. In general, it is used when close margins or microscopically positive margins are suspected. Investigators at Erasmus Medical Center in Rotterdam reported that subjects who had IORT for narrow or microscopically incompletely removed tumors had local control comparable to subjects who had R0 resections close margins.[36,38,39]

At the Mayo Clinic, IORT was used in 52% of subjects with R1 and R2 resections; whereas, it was used in only one-third of the subjects with R0 resection.[13] The investigators reported a 21% and a 27% 5-year survival in subjects who had palliative (R1 and R2) and curative (R0) surgery and IORT, respectively.[13] The pattern of re-recurrence was not described in the study. In a series of 184 consecutive subjects with LRRC, prospectively identified but retrospectively evaluated, where 136 of 147 (92%) subjects undergoing surgical resection for their LRRC received IORT, 57% of the subjects underwent a R0 resection. There were 17 pelvic exenterations and 17 nonanatomic resections. The 30-day mortality was 4.8% and the 90-day mortality was 8.2%. There were 95 complications in 86 subjects (59%). The median overall survival was 28 months. The overall 5-year survival was 32% (48% in R0), with a 34% (52% in R0) 5-year disease-free survival.[25] The local control in this study was reported to be 54% (69% in R0). Multivariate analysis revealed that the only factor significant for local control was radical resection. In terms of survival, the multivariate analysis revealed that the stage of the primary tumor and the radicality of the recurrent surgical procedure were the only statistically significant factors.[25] In this study, approximately 50% of the subjects developed a local re-recurrence or metastatic disease.[25] There was no difference in oncologic outcome between R1 and R2 resections.[25] There was no mention of long-term toxicity secondary to IORT.

From the available data it can be concluded that IORT is a useful adjuvant in the treatment of locally advanced and recurrent rectal cancer for selected patients. However, the surgeon cannot use IORT to supplement an inadequate surgical resection.

RECONSTRUCTION

The empty dead space resulting from extended pelvic resections, such as total pelvic exenterations and abdominosacral resections, predisposes patients to deep abscesses, fistula formation, intestinal obstruction, and perineal wound morbidity. Pelvic floor reconstruction is critical in these patients. A 10-fold increase in wound complications has been reported in patients with a prior history of radiotherapy.[40] Thus, it would be logical to bring well-vascularized tissue to obliterate the dead space and close the perineal wounds. The most common myocutaneous flaps used to close pelvic and perineal defects are the vertical rectus abdominis (VRAM), gracilis, and gluteus maximus.[41] Immediate tissue transfer with a myocutaneous flaps for perineal wound closures have been associated with fewer complications than primary closure in patients undergoing multivisceral resection or prior radiotherapy.[42] Chessin and colleagues[43] reported that the perineal wound complications were significantly less frequent in subjects who underwent myocutaneous flap reconstruction than those with primary closure (16% vs 44%) after neoadjuvant chemoradiation and abdominoperineal resection. Butler and colleagues[44] reported a similar study where there was no significant difference in the incidence of perineal wound complications between those closed primarily and those with myocutaneous flaps. However, in that study, the myocutaneous flap group had a lower incidence of major perineal wound problems, such as abscess, perineal wound dehiscence, and the need for drainage procedures.

There was no significant difference in abdominal wall complications between those subjects who were closed primarily versus those with myocutaneous flaps.[44] The drawback of myocutaneous flaps include the added surgical time and the potential for morbidity.[41] The authors' believe that the potential disadvantages are offset by the potential benefit in patients with recurrent rectal cancer. Thus, the authors' currently use myocutaneous flaps (preferably VRAM) in those patients where extended procedures, such as pelvic exenterations, abdominosacral resection, patient whose perineal skin will be widely resected, and patients who will receive intraoperative radiation. The authors' also favor the use of myocutaneous flaps in those patients who have been previously irradiated and will undergo abdominoperineal resection.

PALLIATION

Palliation for LRRC involves both surgical and nonsurgical therapy. As previously discussed, surgery for LRRC can be a morbid procedure. Palliative pelvic exenterations have been performed to alleviate pelvic pain, tumor-related abscesses, recurrent hemorrhage, bowel obstruction, and entero-urinary or genitourinary fistulas.[45,46] The authors' believe that radical surgical excision (pelvic exenterations) for palliation should be limited to highly selected patients, because leaving the tumor behind will only marginally improve survival, but in some cases improve quality of life. Pain and quality of life after treatment of subjects with LRRC were investigated by Esnaola and colleagues[47] in 45 subjects with locally recurrent rectal cancer at M.D. Anderson Cancer Center. Posttreatment pain severity and QOL were assessed prospectively. Fifteen subjects received nonsurgical palliation of their recurrences; whereas, 30 subjects underwent resection of their recurrence. A significant association between higher posttreatment pain scores and worse quality of life was reported.[47] Subjects treated nonsurgically reported moderate to severe pain beyond the third month of treatment; whereas, those resected had comparable pain during the first 3 postoperative years, particularly after bony resections. However, long-term survivors (>3 years) reported minimal pain and good QOL.[47] The investigators concluded that aggressive pain management after treatment of locally recurrent rectal cancer is warranted as posttreatment pain was pervasive and prolonged.[47]

SUMMARY

Locally recurrent rectal cancer is a complex problem. Patients must be thoroughly evaluated and managed in a multidisciplinary fashion. Chemoradiation, whether external beam or intraoperative radiotherapy, should be considered. Despite all the advances in imaging and surgical techniques, approximately 40% to 60% of patients will achieve a R0 resection. Even though surgical salvage for LRRC is a morbid procedure, long-term survival can be achieved. In highly selected patients, palliative surgical procedures may be performed, but with cautious optimism because palliative surgery may compromise quality of life and, on occasion, may not be better than nonsurgical palliation.

REFERENCES

1. Heald RJ, Moran BJ, Ryall RD, et al. Rectal caner: the Basingstoke experience of total mesorectal excision, 1978–1997. Arch Surg 1998;133:894–8.
2. Sauer R, Becker H, Hohenberger W, et al. Preoperative versus postoperative chemoradiotherapy for rectal cancer. N Engl J Med 2004;351:1731–40.

3. Bedrosian I, Rodriguez-Bigas MA, Feig B, et al. Predicting the node negative mesorectum after preoperative chemoradiation for locally advanced rectal adenocarcinoma. J Gastrointest Surg 2004;8:56–63.
4. Bosset JF, Collette L, Calais G, et al. Chemotherapy with preoperative radiotherapy in rectal cancer. N Engl J Med 2006;355:1114–23.
5. Gerard JP, Conroy T, Bonnetain F, et al. Preoperative radiotherapy with or without concurrent fluorouracil and leucovorin in T3-4 rectal cancers: results of FFCD 9203. J Clin Oncol 2006;24:4620–5.
6. Peeters KC, Marijnen CA, Nagtegaal ID, et al. The TME trial after a median of follow-up of 6 years; increased local control but no survival benefit in irradiated patients with resectable rectal cancer. Ann Surg 2007;246:693–701.
7. Pacelli F, Tortorelli AP, Rosa F, et al. Locally recurrent rectal cancer: prognostic factors and long-term outcomes of multimodal therapy. Ann Surg Oncol 2010; 17:152–62.
8. Bouchard P, Efron J. Management of recurrent rectal cancer. Ann Surg Oncol 2010;17:1343–56.
9. Gunderson LL, Sosin H. Areas of failure found at reoperation (second or symptomatic look) following "curative surgery" for adenocarcinoma of the rectum. Cancer 1974;34(4):1278–92.
10. Suzuki K, Dozois RR, Devine RM, et al. Curative reoperations for locally recurrent rectal cancer. Dis Colon Rectum 1996;39:730–6.
11. Mannaerts GH, Rutten HJ, Martijn H, et al. Comparison of intraoperative radiation therapy-containing multimodality treatment with historical treatment modalities for locally recurrent rectal cancer. Dis Colon Rectum 2001;44:1749–58.
12. Moriya Y. Treatment strategy for locally recurrent rectal cancer. Jpn J Clin Oncol 2006;36:127–31.
13. Hanhloser D, Nelson H, Gunderson LL, et al. Curative potential of multimodality therapy for locally recurrent rectal cancer. Ann Surg 2003;237:502–4.
14. Boyle KM, Sagar PM, Chalmers AG, et al. Surgery for locally recurrent rectal cancer. Dis Colon Rectum 2005;48:929–37.
15. Heriot AG, Byrne CM, Lee P, et al. Extended radical resection the choice for locally recurrent rectal cancer. Dis Colon Rectum 2008;51:284–91.
16. Akasu T, Yamaguchi T, Fujimoto Y, et al. Abdominal sacral resection for posterior pelvic recurrence of rectal carcinoma; analyses of prognostic factors and recurrence patterns. Ann Surg Oncol 2007;14:74–83.
17. Palmer G, Martling A, Cedermark B, et al. A population based study on the management and outcome in patients with locally recurrent rectal cancer. Ann Surg Oncol 2007;14:447–54.
18. Bakx R, Visser O, Josso J, et al. Management of recurrent rectal cancer: a population based study in greater Amsterdam. World J Gastroenterol 2008;14: 6018–23.
19. Paty PB, Nash GM, Baron P, et al. Long-term results of local excision for rectal cancer. Ann Surg 2002;236:522–30.
20. Greenberg JA, Shibata D, Herndon JE II, et al. Local excision of distal rectal cancer: an update of Cancer and Leukemia Group B 8984. Dis Colon Rectum 2008;51:1185–94.
21. Faneyte IF, Dresen RC, Edelbrok MA, et al. Preoperative staging with positron emission tomography in patients with pelvic recurrence of rectal cancer. Dig Surg 2008;25:202–7.
22. Wanebo HJ, Antoniuk P, Koness RJ, et al. Pelvic resection of recurrent rectal cancer: technical considerations. Dis Colon Rectum 1999;42:1438–48.

23. Yamada K, Ishizawa T, Niwa K, et al. Patterns of pelvic invasion are prognostic in the treatment of locally recurrent rectal cancer. Br J Surg 2001;88:988–93.
24. Moore HG, Shoup M, Riedel E, et al. Colorectal cancer pelvic recurrences: determinants of respectability. Dis Colon Rectum 2004;47:1599–606.
25. Dresen RC, Gosens MJ, Martjin H, et al. Radical resection after iort-containing multimodality treatment is the most important determinant for outcome in patients treated for locally recurrent rectal cancer. Ann Surg Oncol 2008;15:1937–47.
26. Pawlik TM, Skibber JM, Rodriguez-Bigas MA. Pelvic exenteration for advanced pelvic malignancies. Ann Surg Oncol 2006;13:612–23.
27. Jimenez R, Shoup M, Cohen A, et al. Contemporary outcomes of total pelvic exenteration in the treatment of colorectal cancer. Dis Colon Rectum 2003;46: 1619–25.
28. Valentini V, Morganti AG, Gambacorta MA, et al. Preoperative hyperfractionated chemoradiation for locally recurrent rectal cancer in patients previously irradiated to the pelvis: a multicentric phase II study. Int J Radiat Oncol Biol Phys 2006;39: 1379–95.
29. Das P, Delclos ME, Skibber JM, et al. Hyperfractionated radiotherapy for rectal cancer in patients with prior irradiation. Int J Radiat Oncol Biol Phys 2010;77:60–5.
30. Mohiuddin M, Marks G, Marks J. Long-term results of reirradiation for patients with recurrent rectal carcinoma. Cancer 2002;95:1144–50.
31. Bedrosian I, Giacco G, Pederson L, et al. Outcome after curative resection for locally recurrent rectal cancer. Dis Colon Rectum 2006;49:175–82.
32. Sagar PM, Gonsalves S, Heath RM, et al. Composite abdominosacral resection for recurrent rectal cancer. Br J Surg 2009;96:191–6.
33. Gunderson LL, Martin JK, Beart RW, et al. Intraoperative and external beam irradiation for locally advanced colorectal cancer. Ann Surg 1988;207:52–60.
34. Rutten HJ, Mannaerts GH, Martijn H, et al. Intraoperative radiotherapy for locally recurrent rectal cancer in The Netherlands. Eur J Surg Oncol 2000;26(Suppl A): s16–20.
35. Azinovic I, Calvo FA, Puebla F, et al. Long –term normal tissue effects of intraoperative electron radiation therapy (IOERT): late sequelae, tumor recurrence, and second malignancies. Int J Radiat Oncol Biol Phys 2001;49:597–604.
36. De Wilt JH, Veermas M, Ferenschild FT, et al. Management of locally advanced primary recurrent rectal cancer. Clin Colon Rectal Surg 2007;20:255–64.
37. Nuyttens JJ, Kolkman-Deurloo IK, Vermaas M, et al. High dose-rate intraoperative radiotherapy for close or positive margins in patients with locally advanced or recurrent rectal cancer. Int J Radiat Oncol Biol Phys 2004;58:106–12.
38. Vermaas M, Ferenschild FT, Nuyttens JJ, et al. Preoperative radiotherapy improves outcomes in recurrent rectal cancer. Dis Colon Rectum 2005;48:918–28.
39. Ferenschild FT, Veermas M, Nuyttens JJ, et al. Value of intraoperative radiotherapy in locally advanced rectal cancer. Dis Colon Rectum 2006;15:71–8.
40. Farid H, O'Connell TX. Methods to decrease the morbidity of abdominoperineal resection. Am Surg 1995;61:1061–4.
41. Butler CE, Rodriguez-Bigas MA. Pelvic reconstruction after abdominoperineal resection is it worthwhile? Ann Surg Oncol 2005;12:91–4.
42. Khoo AK, Skibber JM, Nabawi AS, et al. Indications for immediate tissue transfer for soft tissue reconstruction in pelvic surgery. Surgery 2001;130:463–9.
43. Chessin DB, Hartley J, Cohen AM, et al. Rectus flap reconstruction decreases perineal wound complications following pelvic chemoradiation and surgery: a cohort study. Ann Surg Oncol 2005;12:104–10.

44. Butler CE, Gündeslioglu AO, Rodriguez-Bigas MA. Outcomes of immediate vertical rectus abdominis myocutaneous flap reconstruction for irradiated abdominoperineal resection defects. J Am Coll Surg 2008;206:694–703.
45. Brophy PF, Hoffman JP, Eisenberg BL. The role of palliative pelvic exenteration. Am J Surg 1994;167:386–90.
46. Finlayson CA, Eisenberg BL. Palliative pelvic exenteration: patient selection and results. Oncology (Huntingt) 1996;10:479–84.
47. Esnaola NF, Cantor SB, Johnson ML, et al. Pain and quality of life after treatment in patients with locally recurrent rectal cancer. J Clin Oncol 2002;20:4361–7.

Optimal Follow-Up to Curative Colon and Rectal Cancer Surgery: How and for How Long?

Theodor Asgeirsson, MD[a], Sen Zhang, MD[b],
Anthony J. Senagore, MD, MS, MBA[c],*

KEYWORDS

• Colon cancer • Rectal cancer • Follow-up • Surveillance

In 2009, the projected incidence for colon and rectal cancers in the United States was 106,100 and 40,870, respectively, and approximately 75% of these patients were treated with curative intent. Despite significant improvements in screening and treatment, the 5-year survival ranges from 64% to 90% primarily because of a 30% to 40% incidence of recurrence. Therefore, the annual additional burden of colorectal cancer survivors available for surveillance for recurrence is approximately 110,000 patients.[1,2] Despite significant efforts in refining staging modalities with imaging and even proteogenomics, the American Joint Committee on Cancer (AJCC)/tumor-node-metastasis (TNM) staging system remains the gold standard for recurrence risk stratification. This article attempts to review the current status of the evidence related to surveillance strategies after curative colorectal cancer.

Surveillance or follow-up after colon and rectal cancer resection serves multiple purposes; however, the primary argument supporting the validity of surveillance is the detection of metachronous and recurrent cancers amenable to curative treatment. A secondary benefit is that data from the surveillance protocols provide outcomes-based data for the ongoing assessment of prior, current, and experimental treatment modalities. Finally, the surveillance may provide some comfort for the cancer survivors who can be informed that they have no evidence of disease. There is pressure to

---

[a] Research, Department of Surgery, Spectrum Health, Grand Rapids, MI, USA
[b] Research, Spectrum Health, Grand Rapids, MI, USA
[c] Division of Colon and Rectal Surgery, Department of Colorectal Surgery, Keck School of Medicine, University of Southern California, 1441 Eastlake Avenue, Suite 7418, Los Angeles, CA 90033, USA
* Corresponding author.
E-mail address: anthony.senagore@med.usc.edu

Surg Oncol Clin N Am 19 (2010) 861–873
doi:10.1016/j.soc.2010.06.003
1055-3207/10/$ – see front matter © 2010 Published by Elsevier Inc.

surgonc.theclinics.com

define which surveillance strategies are cost effective. Most of the available data indicate that early identification of recurrent disease at a curative stage may be illusory.[3]

Current guidelines for postoperative follow-up defined by the stakeholder medical societies vary in intensity of evaluation; however, all guidelines focus on a combination of clinical examination, laboratory testing, imaging, and colonoscopy. Despite evaluation of the same evidence-based data, the expert opinions and recommendations can be inconclusive and disparate.[4–6] There are currently (at the time of this article's submission) 8 published randomized trials assessing different regimens for follow-up of patients with colorectal cancer operated for cure.[7–14] Pietra and colleagues[10] reported an increase in 5-year survival (58.3% vs 73.1%; $P<.02$) with intense follow-up aimed at discovering local recurrence for colon and rectal cancer. Local recurrences were significantly more frequent in rectal cancer (36.7%) versus colon cancer (15%), and the survival advantage was likely related to an enhanced opportunity for curative management of those recurrences. The only other randomized controlled trial (RCT) that has demonstrated statistical improvement in survival resulting from intense follow-up was by Rodríguez-Moranta and colleagues.[13] This group assessed stage II and stage III colorectal cancers and reported longer survival in patients with stage II tumor (hazard ratio [HR] = 0.34; 95% confidence interval [CI], 0.12–0.098; $P = .045$) and in those with rectal cancer (HR = 0.09; 95% CI 0.01–0.81; $P = .03$). The investigators' strategy compared a simple surveillance strategy of clinical evaluation and serum carcinoembryonic antigen (CEA) monitoring versus intensive strategy in which abdominal computed tomography (CT) or ultrasonography, chest radiograph, and colonoscopy were added. The remaining studies failed to report statistically significant survival advantage based on studies powered to detect a 15% to 20% survival advantage. The follow-up meta-analyses of these studies similarly failed to confirm a reduction in cancer-related mortality with intense follow-up, although there have been benefits in overall survival and earlier detection of recurrence leading to higher incidence of resections of recurrent disease.[15–17] The recent changes in improved surgical technique and greater use of neoadjuvant and adjuvant chemotherapy and radiation therapy have further confounded the data because of shifts in local and regional failure rates with primary therapy.[18] There are 2 ongoing prospective randomized studies in Europe that may provide clearer information regarding the value of intense surveillance, which are the follow-up after colorectal surgery (FACS) trial and the Gruppo Italiano di Lavoro per la Diagnosi Anticipata (GILDA) trial.[19]

Further complicating the analysis of administrative data sets is not only the diversity of recommendations but also the significant variation in compliance with the recommended surveillance guidelines. A postal survey of active members of the American Society of Colon and Rectal Surgeons (ASCRS) in 2007 demonstrated a wide variation in the frequency of follow-up and the specific diagnostic modalities used. In fact, only 50% of surgeons followed the recommended guidelines as published by the ASCRS. Alternatively, an assessment of follow-up for patients with rectal cancer failed to demonstrate any stage-based differences in patient surveillance strategy.[20,21] Similarly, a survey conducted from the Netherlands of gastrointestinal departments found that 52% of respondents advised shorter interval assessments than advised by national recommendations.[22] This finding was confirmed in a population-based study by Cooper and Doug Kou,[23] which assessed 9426 patients over 12 months and identified significant variation in compliance between geographic areas and race, with 22.7% of patients receiving more investigations than recommended.

There is clearly a significant gap in the evidence to fully guide an appropriate strategy and a set of investigations capable of defining the frequency and duration of surveillance after curative colon and rectal cancer surgery. In the current era of limited resources, there is an urgent need to define a cost-effective strategy that encompasses effective early identification of recurrence while simultaneously limiting cost and complications from evaluation and treatment. One potential area of improvement is enhanced staging and accurate prediction of the potential for recurrence, thus allowing providers to focus on intense surveillance protocols in the highest-risk patients. These components are discussed later in this article.

RISK ASSESSMENT

At this point in time, risk assessment for recurrent colorectal cancer is primarily guided by the initial histopathologic stage and the likely sites for metastatic spread (local, liver, lung). Although various putative molecular markers have been proposed, no formal and validated pattern of genetic alterations has been confirmed.[24] The higher risk of local recurrence for rectal cancer compared with colon cancer has led to imaging strategies for the pelvis, whereas colon cancer imaging strategy focuses on the liver and lung. Most treatment failures occur in the first 24 months after surgical treatment for colorectal cancer, which suggests more intensive early surveillance program. The aggressiveness of surveillance must also be tempered by an assessment of the comorbidities limiting tolerance of reoperation or pharmacologic or radiologic treatment of even minimally recurrent disease. Although palliative chemotherapy or radiation therapy may improve the quality of life and possibly the chance of survival, the identification of this population can be based on symptoms rather than surveillance.

LOCOREGIONAL AND DISTANT RECURRENCE

As mentioned previously, the risk of recurrence increases with advanced primary AJCC/TNM staging, with the highest risk for stage IIb to stage III lesions. The proposed combination of biochemical and imaging modalities is designed to identify locoregional and distant recurrence at a curative stage. Because rectal cancer carries a higher rate of local failure than colon cancer, but with a similar rate of distant metastatic disease, the strategies should be modified for imaging. Another confounder is the absence of data on the impact of adjuvant treatment on timing and pattern of recurrent disease, which may affect the benefit of surveillance and intervention for recurrence. Galandiuk and colleagues[25] evaluated 818 patients (Dukes B2 [stage IIb] and Dukes C [stage III]) managed by 3 different adjuvant treatment protocols and found recurrence rates of 40% for colon and 52% for rectal cancer. The median time to recurrence for all patients was 16.7 months (range 0.5–98 months). Histologic grade and aneuploidy predicted a higher risk of recurrence; however, the timing of recurrence was unaffected. Perforation, adhesion, and invasion to adjacent organs led to earlier recurrence in stage III cancers, whereas adjuvant therapy delayed recurrence but did affect the overall rate of recurrence. Similar findings were noted in a single-institution study by Obrand and Gordon[26] of stage I to III colon and rectal cancers with recurrence rate also related to site of lesion, stage, adjacent visceral invasion, and perforation. The median time to recurrence was 17 months, but ranged from 18 months for local disease to 34 months for distant disease. However, 93% of all recurrences occurred within 48 months from index surgery, indicating a time limit for surveillance. A population-based study on management of colon and rectal recurrences over a 28-year time frame found that over time, there was an increase in 5-year survival of patients older than 75 years that correlated with increase in curative-intent surgery for recurrences of locoregional and metastatic disease ($P<.0001$). The long time frame was biased by significant changes in patient selection for resection for recurrence; however, the rate of surgery for symptomatic recurrence dropped significantly over time (74.9% to 37.5%; $P<.001$). Investigators attributed an increase in 5-year survival to a more favorable stage at the diagnosis of recurrences.[27] Kobayashi and colleagues[28] compared recurrence rates for 5230 colon and rectal cancers and confirmed recurrence risk by stage (I, 3.7%; II, 13.3.%; III, 30.8%: $P<.0001$), and although most recurrences occurred within 3 years (80%) and virtually all recurrences by 5 years (95%), the rate of recurrence was much faster for stage II and III disease, whereas stage I disease was gradual over a 5-year time frame. A German population study raised concerns about the benefit of resection of recurrent disease in a group with a 30.6% rate of recurrence and a 24% rate of R0 resection. Only 2% of patients were alive with no evidence of disease at 2 years after curative re-resection.[2] Harris and colleagues[29] reviewed local recurrences across all stages of colon cancer during a 13-year time frame and reported a 3.1% rate with no primaries at stage I or well differentiated histologically. Once again, tumor fixation, perforation, and fistulization were the primary drivers of local treatment failure in colon cancer, and these features were associated with a short time to recurrence (13 months [range 2–71 months]). Goldberg and colleagues[30] assessed the rate of recurrence for stage II and III recurrences in an adjuvant chemotherapy trial patient population (n = 1247) with 44% of patients recurring; however, 41% of the recurrences had salvage surgery. The patients demonstrated acceptable 5-year, disease-free survival for hepatic, liver, and locoregional recurrences (32%, 27%, and 27%), and postoperative mortality of 2%. Despite an aggressive and expensive intensive follow-up strategy, Goldberg and colleagues reported only a 3.4% absolute increase in cure rate for patients identified during follow-up with either recurrent disease (28 patients) or metachronous lesions (14 patients). Recurrences within the first year from index operation were particularly ominous.

The significant advances in surgical technique and the broader use of neoadjuvant radiation therapy or neoadjuvant chemoradiotherapy have significantly reduced the frequency of local failure in rectal cancer. The Swedish Adjuvant Radiation Trial reported a significant reduction in recurrence with radiotherapy plus surgery versus surgery alone (28% vs 38%; $P<.001$). The benefit was primarily the result of lower local failure (5% vs 13%) rather than distant recurrences (19% vs 14%).[18] Sauer and colleagues[31] reported similar advantages in association with preoperative chemoradiotherapy, and found this approach to be superior to postoperative chemoradiotherapy in terms of complications and local recurrence. These studies also confirmed that rectal cancer recurrence is uncommon after 5 years with or without neoadjuvant therapy. Guillem and colleagues[32] assessed the natural history of locally advanced rectal cancer (T3–4 or N1) after treatment with neoadjuvant chemoradiation and total mesorectal excision (n = 297), and although 23% developed local or distant recurrence, only 1.3% recurred greater than 5 years after surgery. Local failure and survival were affected by pathologic response greater than 95%, lymphovascular invasion, and/or perineural invasion and positive lymph nodes.

METACHRONOUS COLON AND RECTAL NEOPLASMS

Metachronous neoplasms arise from mucosa at a separate site from the primary cancer or anastomosis in a patient with a personal history of previous colon and rectal cancer. Balleste and colleagues[33] in conjunction with the Gastrointestinal Oncology Group of the Spanish Gastrointestinal Association followed 353 patients with colon and rectal cancer for 24 months to define the factors associated with metachronous lesions. All patients had a colonoscopy between years 1 and 2, and the incidence of metachronous neoplasms correlated with familial, pathologic, and molecular characteristics. The incidence of adenomas was 25%, and the metachronous cancer rate was 1.9. Univariate analysis demonstrated that metachronous neoplasms were associated with personal and previous history of colorectal cancer (odds ratio [OR] 5.58; 95% CI 1.01–31.01) and presence of previous or synchronous adenomas (OR 1.77; 95% CI 1.21–3.17). Two large studies have further evaluated metachronous neoplasm rates. The US Multisociety Task Force on Colorectal Cancer reported a 1.5% rate of metachronous cancers amongst 9029 patients, with about half of the lesions occurring within 2 years from initial resection. A French population-based study, which extended over 27 years, reported that long-term risk for metachronous colorectal cancer was 1.8% at 5 years, 3.4% at 10 years, and 7.2% at 20 years, arguing for the value of long-term colonoscopic follow-up in this at-risk population. The existence of a synchronous colorectal cancer also significantly increases the incidence of early-stage metachronous colorectal cancer, which can be managed curatively.[34,35] Therefore, a strategy for adoption of a structured colonoscopic screening program that is focused on eradication of adenomatous polyps may prove to be beneficial. The National Polyp Study demonstrated that patients who have undergone a high-quality colonoscopy with adenoma removal have a very low risk of colon cancer diagnosis at 1 year.[18] This strategy should be applicable to patients surgically managed for colon and rectal cancer, whereby performance of a colonoscopy within 1 to 2 years' postresection should identify any missed synchronous lesions from the index colonoscopy and then allow screening for true metachronous neoplasia.[36] Hyman and colleagues[37] support this contention based on the identification of clinically significant neoplastic lesions found on 1-year follow-up colonoscopy, which occurred primarily in patients who did not have index colonoscopy performed by their operating surgeon. It is unclear whether metachronous cancers actually possess different and more aggressive biologic characteristics as opposed to the possibility of a congenital or acquired increased risk for colonic neoplasia.

COST OF SURVEILLANCE

Health care costs in the United States continue to increase, and a recent article reported a 10.3% annual increase in the cost of surveillance imaging in patients with colorectal cancer from 1999 to 2006.[38] Estimates from the Congressional Budget Office show that the health care spending for an average individual is the highest contributor to increasing health care costs and that the projected spending growth is unsustainable. Every year, 110,000 new patients undergo curative resection of colorectal cancer and become eligible for surveillance. Justification of a surveillance strategy requires evidence of clinical value (identification of recurrence at the point where cure is possible), avoidance of false-positive and false-negative studies, and cost efficiency. Sandler and colleagues[39] presented one of the earliest evaluations of CEA monitoring for 2 years after curative-intent resection. Sandler and colleagues estimated costs of monthly CEA surveillance, assuming a false-negative rate (10%) and false-positive rate (24%), which came to an estimated cost of $24,779 per resectable recurrence. This figure was based on a 2-year recurrence rate of 50% for colon and rectal cancer, and it was rightfully pointed out that the higher the rate of recurrence, the more cost-efficient CEA screening would be. Unfortunately, Sandler and colleagues' CEA strategy could not define whether detection of recurrence truly prolonged life. Transposing their results to modern recurrence rates with earlier stage, more refined surgery, and adjuvant chemotherapy raises even more concerns about the cost of using CEA in isolation. Virgo and colleagues[3] performed an economic analysis of 11 separate surveillance strategies based on Medicare-allowed charges for

5 years of posttreatment follow-up. Virgo and colleagues found a wide range of charges across follow-up strategies, ranging from $910 to $26,717, with no clear evidence that higher-cost strategies increased survival or quality of life. In the late 1990s, Kievit and Bruinvels[40] presented results of a cost-effectiveness analysis used to model the natural history of colon and rectal cancer recurrence comparing no follow-up, selective follow-up, and intensive follow-up. In a simulated trial of 3 × 20,000 patients, follow-up provided no increase in quality-adjusted life years, but cost estimates increased 1.65 times from selective to intense follow-up (Dfl.6190 ± 3170 and 7450 ± 3330), and no marginal cost-effectiveness of the follow-up scenarios tested was below the acceptable range of Dfl.50,000 per quality-adjusted life year gained. Sensitivity analysis suggested that older age and favorable TNM stage decreases effectiveness of colorectal cancer follow-up. The investigators question whether the curability of colorectal cancer recurrences is a time-dependent phenomenon, and because no clear evidence points to increased survival for earlier resection or resection of asymptomatic recurrences, the justification of intense follow-up may not only be costly but also may not be clearly tied to the desired outcomes. The first study to examine the relative and absolute costs of physical examination, CEA, chest radiograph, and colonoscopy in detecting recurrent disease after Dukes B2 or Dukes C was published by Graham and colleagues[41] in 1998. Clinical examination failed to identify a single resectable recurrence but was associated with a total cost of $418,615. The detection rate for CEA was 2.2%; chest radiograph 0.9%; colonoscopy 1%; and the respective cost per recurrence was $5696, $10,078, and $45,810. The investigators determined that CEA was the most cost-effective test in detecting potentially curable recurrent disease. Of the 1356 patients reviewed, only 14 (1%) were identified who were both asymptomatic and amenable to a potentially curative resection. The investigators did not report the long-term survival of the patients. Collective evidence has shown that efficacy of colon and rectal cancer follow-up is between 2% and 5%, which implies that more than 90% of patients followed have no direct benefit from follow-up. Staib and colleagues[42] looked at the cost-effectiveness in 1054 patients of all stages of colon and rectal cancer over 10 years of follow-up, which included quarterly visits in the first 2 years, biannual visits in years 3 to 5, and subsequent yearly visits in years 6 to 10. Laboratory tests were performed with all visits, but imaging and endoscopy were limited to the first 5 years of follow-up (ultrasonography, chest radiograph, colonoscopy, and pelvis CT for rectal cancers). The follow-up costs for 21 cured recurrences were €126,000, resulting in a cost-effectiveness of 50:1 and efficacy of 2%. With these results, the investigators emphasize that tests performed should be based on sensitivity and specificity. Risk-adjusted follow-up should focus on high-risk patients for 2 to 3 years to increase cost efficiency. Bleeker and colleagues[43] looked at the value and cost of follow-up after adjuvant treatment of patients with Dukes C colon cancer (n = 496) and found that most recurrences were identified by liver ultrasonography or CT, and the mean cost of diagnostic procedures per curative resected recurrence was $9011. Ultrasonography and colonoscopy identified 22 recurrences at a cost of $11,790 per patient, whereas CEA, chest radiograph, and physical examination identified a further 6 recurrences at a cost of $19,850. These findings are somewhat contradictory to previous publications on the cost effectiveness of CEA in surveillance but can be explained by the fact that 30% of colorectal cancers do not produce CEA, and even lesions that secrete CEA require additional localizing studies to assess potential respectability.[41] A stage-based, Markov simulation model assessment of cost effectiveness revealed good results for Dukes C patients (a ratio of €1058 [±2746] per quality of life years compared with a simplified follow-up), but was less favorable when Dukes A and Dukes B ratios were calculated.[44]

CURRENT GUIDELINES

Published guidelines from 3 subspecialty groups are summarized in **Table 1**. All societies recommend some form of follow-up based on their individual assessments of the same data available in the literature. As mentioned previously, and supported by all 3 societies, colonoscopy is an important part of follow-up after colon and rectal cancer resection for the detection of metachronous colorectal neoplasms. After a normal postoperative colonoscopy to exclude missed synchronous lesions, a surveillance examination every 3 years seems reasonable.

ASCRS recommendations were based primarily on 2 meta-analyses that included 5 RCTs comparing the intensity of follow-up and concluded that a survival advantage was associated with a more intense strategy.[15,45] ASCRS guidelines state that despite the fact that 16% to 66% of recurrences present with symptoms, the role of clinical examination seems very limited.[46] ASCRS recommends quarterly CEA measurement for 2 years, because elevation of greater than 5 ng/mL has a positive predictive value of 70% to 80% and has a 4- to 6-month lead time for recurrence compared with other available tests.[47] ASCRS does not recommend routine use of hepatic imaging in the follow-up of colon and rectal cancer, and cannot support or refute routine use of chest radiograph based on available data. Ultrasonography and CT have a reported sensitivity of 60% and 75%, respectively, and options for treatment of metastasis have increased during the last 30 years, resulting in 5-year survival of around 30% after metasectomy.[48] Despite these advances and moderate rates of detection, published data on hepatic imaging in follow-up lead to resection of disease in only 1.3% to 1.8% of patients followed.[11,49] The identification of resectable disease with chest radiograph is low (0.9%–12%),[50,51] and there are no studies that have looked at survival using chest radiograph as a surveillance modality.

The American Society of Clinical Oncology (ASCO) updated guidelines from 2005 similarly refer to meta-analysis that reported a 20% to 33% reduction (7% absolute risk reduction) in the risk of death from all causes for patients who received intensive follow-up, although only 2 out of 6 RCTs suggested significant improvement with intensive follow-up.[10,12,15,45,52] ASCO justifies clinical examination primarily based on the construct that the patient-doctor interaction may affect assessment of risk and detection of asymptomatic recurrences, which may allow for genetic testing and addressing patient queries. However, ASCO cannot confirm a survival effect of this strategy. ASCO states that serum CEA testing should be performed for patients with stage II or stage III if the patient is a candidate for surgery or systemic therapy and an elevation warrants retesting to confirm a rising level.[53] Testing should be evaluated carefully during treatment, because fluorouracil-based therapy may falsely elevate CEA.[54,55] ASCO recommends CT of the chest and abdomen yearly for 3 years for patients at high risk of recurrence, who are candidates for resection. A pelvic CT should be considered for rectal cancer surveillance for candidates who have not been treated with radiotherapy.

The Association of Coloproctology of Great Britain and Ireland (ACPGBI) points out the discrepancies between published RCTs in intensity of follow-up and the low statistical power of these studies. This group has recommended a more conservative approach and states that current data have not clearly shown a significant effect on survival despite that the benefit may accrue to a more intense strategy has not been refuted. There does seem to be some data suggesting that earlier detection of recurrent disease may improve quality of life with current modalities of chemotherapy and that a small number of patients may actually be cured.[56,57] The ACPGBI supports office follow-up without a defined interval or frequency, primarily to provide patient support and surgical audit. However, the ACPGBI suggests this role may be delegated to specialized nursing staff to reduce

Table 1
Current surveillance guidelines for colon and rectal cancer from 3 specialty societies: the ASCRS, the American Society of Clinical Oncology (ASCO), and the Association of Coloproctology of Great Britain and Ireland (ACPGBI)

	ASCRS[5]	ASCO[6]	ACPGBI[62]
Office visit	3 times per year for 2 y	3–6 mo for 2 y, then 6 mo for year 4–5	Audit mandated but no recommendation for frequency
Laboratory test	CEA 3 times per year for 2 y	CEA 4 times per year for 3 y or longer for patients with stage II or stage III	Not recommended
Imaging	Not recommended	CT chest and abdomen yearly for 3 y. Consider CT pelvis for rectal cancer if no radiation	Liver and chest imaging (ultrasonography or CT) within 2 y of resection for asymptomatic patients
Colonoscopy	Every 3 y	At 3 y and then every 5 y if normal	Every 3–5 y

costs.[58] ACPGBI does not recommend CEA monitoring because of the limited impact on survival when comparing the work by Pietra and colleagues[10] (only trial with benefit) and 2 additional publications with no benefit.[12,59] The ACPGBI makes a similar argument to ASCRS; however, a different conclusion was reached with respect to liver and chest imaging within 2 years from resection in asymptomatic individuals. Pietra and colleagues argue that imaging improves the likelihood of being able to offer potentially curative hepatic resection in less than 5% of patients.

SUMMARY, CURRENT CHALLENGES, AND FUTURE DIRECTIONS

There is a modest amount of solid evidence-based guidance regarding the role of surveillance after curative colon and rectal cancer. In particular, the case for cost-effective intense surveillance leading to improved survival remains elusive. The most recent meta-analysis by Tjandra and Chan,[16] which included 8 RCTs with 2923 colorectal cancers, found a statistically significant reduction in overall mortality with intense follow-up (21.8 vs 25.7%; $P = .01$); however, this represents an absolute reduction in mortality of less than 4%. CEA ($P = .00020$) and colonoscopy ($P = .04$) demonstrated a significant impact on survival; however, the cancer-related mortality did not improve with earlier detection and treatment of recurrent disease. The Cochrane Collaborative review by Jeffery and colleagues[17] also concluded that a survival benefit accrued to patients undergoing more intensive follow-up. There was a mortality benefit associated with performing more tests versus fewer and with liver imaging versus no liver imaging. However, this strategy led to more surgical procedures attempted for cure in the intensively followed arm, and the morbidity and mortality impact were not assessed. In addition, the investigators could not identify a specific battery of tests that are helpful. Therefore, one must be aware that although meta-analysis may represent level I evidence, the validity is limited by the underlying quality of the RCTs on which they are based. Overreliance on flawed data can lead to clinical patterns that may be detrimental.[60] There are 2 RCTs currently accruing patients that may shed some light on the effectiveness of surveillance. The Italian GILDA trial attempts to compare intense versus minimal follow-up for Dukes B and Dukes C with a projected accrual of 2929 patients. The aim is to define overall survival, colorectal cancer mortality, quality of life, and time to detection of recurrence. The United Kingdom FACS trial is comparing primary care follow-up with CEA versus intense specialist-based follow-up with CT and ultrasound scanning, and attempts to randomize 4890 patients. Similar outcomes to the GILDA trial are monitored in addition to the detection and treatment of metastatic disease by a multidisciplinary team of surgeons and medical oncologists capable of managing multivisceral metastatic disease.

We clearly must strive to improve the quality of data based on accurate risk stratification of recurrence risk and early identification of recurrent disease when curative intervention is possible, and provide a value-based strategy within the current economic constraints faced by medical systems. We must improve on the analysis by Ohlsson and Palsson,[61] who calculated the proportion of patients that might benefit from follow-up based on efficacy of available data. Out of 100 patients resected for cure, 33 develop recurrence with 7 qualifying for re-resection and 3 actually cured (3000 patients cured out of 100,000 who potentially are enrolled in surveillance yearly in the United States).

REFERENCES

1. Smith RA, Cokkinides V, Brawley OW. Cancer screening in the United States, 2009: a review of current American Cancer Society guidelines and issues in cancer screening. CA Cancer J Clin 2009;59(1):27–41.

2. Bohm B, Schwenk W, Hucke HP, et al. Does methodic long-term follow-up affect survival after curative resection of colorectal carcinoma? Dis Colon Rectum 1993; 36(3):280–6.
3. Virgo KS, Vernava AM, Longo WE, et al. Cost of patient follow-up after potentially curative colorectal cancer treatment. JAMA 1995;273(23):1837–41.
4. Lee PW. ACPGBI annual meeting. Colorectal Dis 2001;3(4):276–8.
5. Anthony T, Simmang C, Hyman N, et al. Practice parameters for the surveillance and follow-up of patients with colon and rectal cancer. Dis Colon Rectum 2004; 47(6):807–17.
6. Desch CE, Benson AB 3rd, Somerfield MR, et al. Colorectal cancer surveillance: 2005 update of an American Society of Clinical Oncology practice guideline. J Clin Oncol 2005;23(33):8512–9.
7. Makela JT, Laitinen SO, Kairaluoma MI. Five-year follow-up after radical surgery for colorectal cancer. Results of a prospective randomized trial. Arch Surg 1995; 130(10):1062–7.
8. Ohlsson B, Breland U, Ekberg H, et al. Follow-up after curative surgery for colorectal carcinoma. Randomized comparison with no follow-up. Dis Colon Rectum 1995;38(6):619–26.
9. Kjeldsen BJ, Kronborg O, Fenger C, et al. A prospective randomized study of follow-up after radical surgery for colorectal cancer. Br J Surg 1997;84(5):666–9.
10. Pietra N, Sarli L, Costi R, et al. Role of follow-up in management of local recurrences of colorectal cancer: a prospective, randomized study. Dis Colon Rectum 1998;41(9):1127–33.
11. Schoemaker D, Black R, Giles L, et al. Yearly colonoscopy, liver CT, and chest radiography do not influence 5-year survival of colorectal cancer patients. Gastroenterology 1998;114(1):7–14.
12. Secco GB, Fardelli R, Gianquinto D, et al. Efficacy and cost of risk-adapted follow-up in patients after colorectal cancer surgery: a prospective, randomized and controlled trial. Eur J Surg Oncol 2002;28(4):418–23.
13. Rodríguez-Moranta F, Saló J, Arcusa A, et al. Postoperative surveillance in patients with colorectal cancer who have undergone curative resection: a prospective, multicenter, randomized, controlled trial. J Clin Oncol 2006;24(3):386–93.
14. Wattchow DA, Weller DP, Esterman A, et al. General practice vs surgical-based follow-up for patients with colon cancer: randomised controlled trial. Br J Cancer 2006;94(8):1116–21.
15. Renehan AG, Egger M, Saunders MP, et al. Impact on survival of intensive follow-up after curative resection for colorectal cancer: systematic review and meta-analysis of randomised trials. BMJ 2002;324(7341):813.
16. Tjandra JJ, Chan MK. Follow-up after curative resection of colorectal cancer: a meta-analysis. Dis Colon Rectum 2007;50(11):1783–99.
17. Jeffery M, Hickey BE, Hider PN. Follow-up strategies for patients treated for non-metastatic colorectal cancer. Cochrane Database Syst Rev 2007;1:CD002200.
18. Improved survival with preoperative radiotherapy in resectable rectal cancer. Swedish rectal cancer trial. N Engl J Med 1997;336(14):980–7.
19. Grossmann EM, Johnson FE, Virgo KS, et al. Follow-up of colorectal cancer patients after resection with curative intent-the GILDA trial. Surg Oncol 2004; 13(2–3):119–24.
20. Giordano P, Efron J, Vernava AM 3rd, et al. Strategies of follow-up for colorectal cancer: a survey of the American Society of Colon and Rectal Surgeons. Tech Coloproctol 2006;10(3):199–207.

21. Ode K, Patel U, Virgo KS, et al. How initial tumor stage affects rectal cancer patient follow-up. Oncol Rep 2009;21(6):1511–7.
22. Mulder SA, Ouwendijk RJ, van Leerdam ME, et al. A nationwide survey evaluating adherence to guidelines for follow-up after polypectomy or treatment for colorectal cancer. J Clin Gastroenterol 2008;42(5):487–92.
23. Cooper GS, Doug Kou T. Underuse of colorectal cancer screening in a cohort of Medicare beneficiaries. Cancer 2008;112(2):293–9.
24. Crawford NP, Colliver DW, Galandiuk S. Tumor markers and colorectal cancer: utility in management. J Surg Oncol 2003;84(4):239–48.
25. Galandiuk S, Wieand HS, Moertel CG, et al. Patterns of recurrence after curative resection of carcinoma of the colon and rectum. Surg Gynecol Obstet 1992; 174(1):27–32.
26. Obrand DI, Gordon PH. Incidence and patterns of recurrence following curative resection for colorectal carcinoma. Dis Colon Rectum 1997;40(1):15–24.
27. Guyot F, Faivre J, Manfredi S, et al. Time trends in the treatment and survival of recurrences from colorectal cancer. Ann Oncol 2005;16(5):756–61.
28. Kobayashi H, Ueno H, Hashiguchi Y, et al. Distribution of lymph node metastasis is a prognostic index in patients with stage III colon cancer. Surgery 2006;139(4): 516–22.
29. Harris GJ, Church JM, Senagore AJ, et al. Factors affecting local recurrence of colonic adenocarcinoma. Dis Colon Rectum 2002;45(8):1029–34.
30. Goldberg RM, Fleming TR, Tangen CM, et al. Surgery for recurrent colon cancer: strategies for identifying resectable recurrence and success rates after resection. Eastern Cooperative Oncology Group, the North Central Cancer Treatment Group, and the Southwest Oncology Group. Ann Intern Med 1998; 129(1):27–35.
31. Sauer R, Becker H, Hohenberger W, et al. Preoperative versus postoperative chemoradiotherapy for rectal cancer. N Engl J Med 2004;351(17):1731–40.
32. Guillem JG, Moore HG, Akhurst T, et al. Sequential preoperative fluorodeoxyglucose-positron emission tomography assessment of response to preoperative chemoradiation: a means for determining long-term outcomes of rectal cancer. J Am Coll Surg 2004;199(1):1–7.
33. Balleste B, Bessa X, Pinol V, et al. Detection of metachronous neoplasms in colorectal cancer patients: identification of risk factors. Dis Colon Rectum 2007;50(7): 971–80.
34. Rex DK, Kahi CJ, Levin B, et al. Guidelines for colonoscopy surveillance after cancer resection: a consensus update by the American Cancer Society and the US Multi-Society Task Force on Colorectal Cancer. Gastroenterology 2006; 130(6):1865–71.
35. Bouvier AM, Latournerie M, Jooste V, et al. The lifelong risk of metachronous colorectal cancer justifies long-term colonoscopic follow-up. Eur J Cancer 2008; 44(4):522–7.
36. Pabby A, Schoen RE, Weissfeld JL, et al. Analysis of colorectal cancer occurrence during surveillance colonoscopy in the dietary polyp prevention trial. Gastrointest Endosc 2005;61(3):385–91.
37. Hyman N, Moore J, Cataldo P, et al. The high yield of 1-year colonoscopy after resection: is it the handoff? Surg Endosc 2010;24(3):648–52.
38. Dinan MA, Curtis LH, Hammill BG, et al. Changes in the use and costs of diagnostic imaging among Medicare beneficiaries with cancer, 1999–2006. JAMA 2010;303(16):1625–31.

39. Sandler RS, Freund DA, Herbst CA Jr, et al. Cost effectiveness of postoperative carcinoembryonic antigen monitoring in colorectal cancer. Cancer 1984;53(1): 193–8.
40. Kievit J, Bruinvels DJ. Detection of recurrence after surgery for colorectal cancer. Eur J Cancer Am 1995;31(7–8):1222–5.
41. Graham RA, Wang S, Catalano PJ, et al. Postsurgical surveillance of colon cancer: preliminary cost analysis of physician examination, carcinoembryonic antigen testing, chest x-ray, and colonoscopy. Ann Surg 1998;228(1):59–63.
42. Staib L, Link KH, Beger HG. Follow-up in colorectal cancer: cost-effectiveness analysis of established and novel concepts. Langenbecks Arch Surg 2000; 385(6):412–20.
43. Bleeker WA, Mulder NH, Hermans J, et al. Value and cost of follow-up after adjuvant treatment of patients with Dukes' C colonic cancer. Br J Surg 2001;88(1): 101–6.
44. Borie F, Combescure C, Daures JP, et al. Cost-effectiveness of two follow-up strategies for curative resection of colorectal cancer: comparative study using a Markov model. World J Surg 2004;28(6):563–9.
45. Jeffery GM, Hickey BE, Hider P. Follow-up strategies for patients treated for non-metastatic colorectal cancer. Cochrane Database Syst Rev 2002;1:CD002200.
46. McCredie M, Macfarlane GJ, Bell J, et al. Second primary cancers after cancers of the colon and rectum in New South Wales, Australia, 1972–1991. Cancer Epidemiol Biomarkers Prev 1997;6(3):155–60.
47. McCall JL, Black RB, Rich CA, et al. The value of serum carcinoembryonic antigen in predicting recurrent disease following curative resection of colorectal cancer. Dis Colon Rectum 1994;37(9):875–81.
48. Fong Y, Cohen AM, Fortner JG, et al. Liver resection for colorectal metastases. J Clin Oncol 1997;15(3):938–46.
49. Howell JD, Wotherspoon H, Leen E, et al. Evaluation of a follow-up programme after curative resection for colorectal cancer. Br J Cancer 1999;79(2):308–10.
50. Peethambaram P, Weiss M, Loprinzi CL, et al. An evaluation of postoperative follow-up tests in colon cancer patients treated for cure. Oncology 1997;54(4): 287–92.
51. Abir F, Alva S, Longo WE, et al. The postoperative surveillance of patients with colon cancer and rectal cancer. Am J Surg 2006;192(1):100–8.
52. Figueredo A, Rumble RB, Maroun J, et al. Follow-up of patients with curatively resected colorectal cancer: a practice guideline. BMC Cancer 2003;3:26.
53. Safi F, Beyer HG. The value of follow-up after curative surgery of colorectal carcinoma. Cancer Detect Prev 1993;17(3):417–24.
54. Fletcher RH. Carcinoembryonic antigen. Ann Intern Med 1986;104(1):66–73.
55. Moertel CG, Fleming TR, Macdonald JS, et al. An evaluation of the carcinoembryonic antigen (CEA) test for monitoring patients with resected colon cancer. JAMA 1993;270(8):943–7.
56. Rees M, Plant G, Bygrave S. Late results justify resection for multiple hepatic metastases from colorectal cancer. Br J Surg 1997;84(8):1136–40.
57. Expectancy or primary chemotherapy in patients with advanced asymptomatic colorectal cancer: a randomized trial. J Clin Oncol 1992;10(6):904–11.
58. Jeyarajah S, Adams K, Higgins L, et al. Prospective evaluation of a Colorectal Cancer Nurse Follow-up Clinic. Colorectal Dis 2009. [Epub ahead of print].
59. Northover J, Houghton J, Lennon T. CEA to detect recurrence of colon cancer. JAMA 1994;272(1):31.

60. Devereaux PJ, Bhandari M, Clarke M, et al. Need for expertise based randomised controlled trials. BMJ 2005;330(7482):88.

61. Ohlsson B, Palsson B. Follow-up after colorectal cancer surgery. Acta Oncol 2003;42(8):816–26.

62. Ireland TAoCoGBa. Guidelines for the management of colorectal cancer 3rd edition (2007). Available at: http://www.acpgbi.org.uk/assets/documents/COLO_guides.pdf. 2007. Accessed June 17, 2010.

Index

Note: Page numbers of article titles are in **boldface** type.

Surg Oncol Clin N Am 19 (2010) 875–885
doi:10.1016/S1055-3207(10)00075-X
1055-3207/10/$ – see front matter © 2010 Elsevier Inc. All rights reserved.

surgonc.theclinics.com

Moving?

Make sure your subscription moves with you!

To notify us of your new address, find your **Clinics Account Number** (located on your mailing label above your name), and contact customer service at:

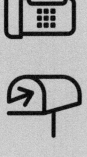

Email: journalscustomerservice-usa@elsevier.com

800-654-2452 (subscribers in the U.S. & Canada)
314-447-8871 (subscribers outside of the U.S. & Canada)

Fax number: 314-447-8029

Elsevier Health Sciences Division
Subscription Customer Service
3251 Riverport Lane
Maryland Heights, MO 63043

ELSEVIER

United States Postal Service

Statement of Ownership, Management, and Circulation
(All Periodicals Publications Except Requestor Publications)

1. Publication Title	2. Publication Number	3. Filing Date
Surgical Oncology Clinics of North America	0 1 2 - 5 6 5	9/15/10

4. Issue Frequency	5. Number of Issues Published Annually	6. Annual Subscription Price
Jan, Apr, Jul, Oct	4	$225.00

7. Complete Mailing Address of Known Office of Publication (Not printer) (Street, city, county, state, and ZIP+4®)

Elsevier Inc.
360 Park Avenue South
New York, NY 10010-1710

Contact Person
Stephen Bushing
Telephone (Include area code)
215-239-3688

8. Complete Mailing Address of Headquarters or General Business Office of Publisher (Not printer)

Elsevier Inc., 360 Park Avenue South, New York, NY 10010-1710

9. Full Names and Complete Mailing Addresses of Publisher, Editor, and Managing Editor (Do not leave blank)

Publisher (Name and complete mailing address)

Kim Murphy, Elsevier, Inc., 1600 John F. Kennedy Blvd. Suite 1800, Philadelphia, PA 19103-2899

Editor (Name and complete mailing address)

Jessica Demetriou, Elsevier, Inc., 1600 John F. Kennedy Blvd. Suite 1800, Philadelphia, PA 19103-2899

Managing Editor (Name and complete mailing address)

Jessica Demetriou, Elsevier, Inc., 1600 John F. Kennedy Blvd. Suite 1800, Philadelphia, PA 19103-2899

10. Owner (Do not leave blank. If the publication is owned by a corporation, give the name and address of the corporation immediately followed by the names and addresses of all stockholders owning or holding 1 percent or more of the total amount of stock. If not owned by a corporation, give the names and addresses of the individual owners. If owned by a partnership or other unincorporated firm, give its name and address as well as those of each individual owner. If the publication is published by a nonprofit organization, give its name and address.)

Full Name	Complete Mailing Address
Wholly owned subsidiary of	4520 East-West Highway
Reed/Elsevier, US holdings	Bethesda, MD 20814

11. Known Bondholders, Mortgagees, and Other Security Holders Owning or Holding 1 Percent or More of Total Amount of Bonds, Mortgages, or Other Securities. If none, check box. ☐ None

Full Name	Complete Mailing Address
N/A	

12. Tax Status (For completion by nonprofit organizations authorized to mail at nonprofit rates) (Check one)
The purpose, function, and nonprofit status of this organization and the exempt status for federal income tax purposes:
☐ Has Not Changed During Preceding 12 Months
☐ Has Changed During Preceding 12 Months (Publisher must submit explanation of change with this statement)

PS Form 3526, September 2007 (Page 1 of 3 (Instructions Page 3)) PSN 7530-01-000-9931 PRIVACY NOTICE: See our Privacy policy in www.usps.com

---

13. Publication Title	14. Issue Date for Circulation Data Below
Surgical Oncology Clinics of North America	July 2010

15. Extent and Nature of Circulation			Average No. Copies Each Issue During Preceding 12 Months	No. Copies of Single Issue Published Nearest to Filing Date
a. Total Number of Copies (Net press run)			864	860
b. Paid Circulation (By Mail and Outside the Mail)	(1)	Mailed Outside-County Paid Subscriptions Stated on PS Form 3541. (Include paid distribution above nominal rate, advertiser's proof copies, and exchange copies)	288	296
	(2)	Mailed In-County Paid Subscriptions Stated on PS Form 3541 (Include paid distribution above nominal rate, advertiser's proof copies, and exchange copies)		
	(3)	Paid Distribution Outside the Mails Including Sales Through Dealers and Carriers, Street Vendors, Counter Sales, and Other Paid Distribution Outside USPS®	155	160
	(4)	Paid Distribution by Other Classes Mailed Through the USPS (e.g. First-Class Mail®)		
c. Total Paid Distribution (Sum of 15b (1), (2), (3), and (4))		▶	443	456
d. Free or Nominal Rate Distribution (By Mail and Outside the Mail)	(1)	Free or Nominal Rate Outside-County Copies Included on PS Form 3541	57	56
	(2)	Free or Nominal Rate In-County Copies Included on PS Form 3541		
	(3)	Free or Nominal Rate Copies Mailed at Other Classes Through the USPS (e.g. First-Class Mail)		
	(4)	Free or Nominal Rate Distribution Outside the Mail (Carriers or other means)		
e. Total Free or Nominal Rate Distribution (Sum of 15d (1), (2), (3) and (4))		▶	57	56
f. Total Distribution (Sum of 15c and 15e)		▶	500	512
g. Copies not Distributed (See instructions to publishers #4 (page #3))		▶	364	348
h. Total (Sum of 15f and g)		▶	864	860
i. Percent Paid (15c divided by 15f times 100)			88.60%	89.06%

16. Publication of Statement of Ownership
☐ If the publication is a general publication, publication of this statement is required. Will be printed in the October 2010 issue of this publication. ☐ Publication not required.

17. Signature and Title of Editor, Publisher, Business Manager, or Owner

Stephen R. Bushing   Date: September 15, 2010

Stephen R. Bushing – Fulfillment/Inventory Specialist

I certify that all information furnished on this form is true and complete. I understand that anyone who furnishes false or misleading information on this form or who omits material or information requested on the form may be subject to criminal sanctions (including fines and imprisonment) and/or civil sanctions (including civil penalties).

PS Form 3526, September 2007 (Page 2 of 3)

Printed and bound by CPI Group (UK) Ltd, Croydon, CR0 4YY

03/10/2024

01040449-0018